CW00455194

© Copyright 2020 by Amina Subramani & Tracy Cooper.

All rights reserved.

This document is geared towards providing exact and reliable information with regard to the topic and issue covered. The publication is sold with the idea that the publisher is not required to render accounting, officially permitted, or otherwise, qualified services. If advice is necessary legal or professional, a practiced individual in the profession should be bordered.

-From a Declaration of Principles which was accepted and approved equally by a Committee of the American Bar Association and a Committee of Publishers and Associations.

In no way is it legal to reproduce, duplicate, or transmit any part of this document in either electronic means or in printed format. Recording of this publication is strictly prohibited and any storage of this document is not allowed unless with written permission from the publisher.

All rights reserved.

The information provided herein is stated to be truthful and consistent, in that any liability, in terms of inattention or otherwise, by any usage or abuse of any policies, processes, or directions contained within is the solitary and utter responsibility of the recipient reader. Under no circumstances will any legal responsibility or blame be held against the publisher for any reparation, damages, or monetary loss due to the information herein, either directly or indirectly.

Respective authors own all copyrights not held by the publisher. The information herein is offered for informational purposes solely and is universal as so. The presentation of the information is without a contract or any type of guarantee assurance.

The trademarks that are used are without any consent, and the publication of the trademark is without permission or backing by the trademark owner. All trademarks and brands within this book are for clarifying purposes only and are owned by the owners themselves, not affiliated with this document.

TABLE OF CONTENTS

INTRODUCTION

SECOND COURSE

MAIN COURSE

DESSERTS & SNACKS

DRINKS & SMOOTHIES

Introduction: (by researcher Mrs. Tracy Copper)

The anti-inflammatory diet is designed to prevent or effectively counteract the risk of inflammation. Therefore, it is not to be considered as a simple slimming cure or any latest fashion diet, but more as a diet that facilitates the body in proper self-defense from the aforementioned inflammations. Although drugs and medical treatments are certainly important, many experts say that following an anti-inflammatory diet would be equally helpful. If you suffer from some type of pathology that as a consequence leads to inflammation, being more attentive to your lifestyle and changing the dietary pattern and eating habits according to your needs, are decisive choices for the health and general well-being of your body. Of course, suddenly changing what we choose to serve at the table will not be the equivalent of a stroke of a magic wand that solves all the problems, but it is certainly a good starting point.

What is the Anti-Inflammatory Diet?

First, let's spend a few words to understand what inflammation is: Inflammation is a condition that can chronically affect each of us, and which is associated with premature aging and numerous other disorders. To combat it, it can be useful to resort to the anti-inflammatory diet, a real ally of health! Inflammation consists of a set of processes by which the body reacts to the action of harmful agents, such as bacteria or viruses, or to the external or internal damage it may encounter. Normally, the inflammation resolves after a few days, following the restoration of damaged tissues and the body's predisposition to complete healing. However, the inflammation may become chronic, condemning those who suffer from it to continuous fluctuations in intensity and duration. Moments when the pain is bearable or almost imperceptible alternate with moments when it becomes difficult to even perform the most common movements. Imagine the discomfort of those who have to live forever with gastritis or arthritis, common manifestations of chronic inflammation, as are Crohn's disease or ulcerative colitis in the intestine. In these cases, in addition to the doctor's advice, who will prescribe the right therapy for each of these disorders, nutrition can also play a fundamental role.

Some foods have strong anti-inflammatory properties, which it would be useful to include in your diet, and foods that should be avoided. Even the number of calories we introduce each day can become an aggravating factor of inflammation, especially when energy consumption does not justify its introduction. Eating more than we need is never a good idea. The anti-inflammatory diet is a dietary regimen recommended to combat some pathological conditions of the body such as arthritis or psoriasis. What are the primary foods that characterize this diet? Green fruit and vegetables, preferably fresh and in season, whole grains (barley, spelled, wheat, and brown rice), extra virgin olive oil, fish rich in omega 3, flax seeds, and some spices like turmeric. Among the foods to be preferred, also legumes, soy, and nuts as well as a good supply of liquids (water, tea, and herbal teas).

What cooking does the anti-inflammatory diet provide?

For even higher quality, the ideal would be to consume foods grown organically, to the detriment of those found in large retailers. In addition to varying the food every day, you prefer genuine cooking such as boiling or grilling.

How does it work?

Inflammation is a natural process that generally helps the body defend itself against infections, diseases, and injuries. We will all have surely had to deal with the banalest symptoms of an infection, such as pain, fever, burning, and so on, but if the aforementioned inflammation is chronic, it means that it acts in our body in a silent and above all destructive, triggering a series of pathologies that can cause quite serious health problems. Chronic inflammation can last for weeks, months, or even years, and has become a very common pathological condition, mainly due to a stressful lifestyle as well as a lack of physical exercise. Given that our choices in terms of nutrition can influence the levels of inflammation in our body, the anti-inflammatory diet is precisely designed to contain inflammation. The typical anti-inflammatory diet favors the intake of alkalizing foods, fiber, and omega 3 acids, while it is necessary to reduce the intake of simple sugars, salt and above all saturated fats, all making sure to receive the right dose of vitamins, minerals, and water. Let's see more precisely which foods it is good to favor and which ones to avoid.

FOODS TO EAT AND AVOID

FOODS TO INCLUDE:

To stick to the type of anti-inflammatory diet it is essential to include anti-inflammatory foods starting primarily with fruits and vegetables, choosing green leafy vegetables rich in beneficial nutrients and a source of vitamin K such as spinach, broccoli, and kale. The berries are in turn full of vitamins and minerals but, more importantly, they contain vegetable pigments called anthocyanins, which is the substance that gives them the typical color of berries and that helps to combat inflammation and reduce the risk. of heart disease. Dried fruit is also for us, thanks to the high content of good fats that help stop inflammation, but always without overdoing the portions. Speaking of good fats, we can find plenty of them in avocado, now a very famous and versatile fruit, but above all in extra-virgin olive oil and cold-pressed linseed oil. Another inevitable food in an anti-inflammatory diet is above all fish, try to eat it at least twice a week, preferring salmon, tuna, sardines, and mackerel, all with omega 3 acids which, as already mentioned, are essential to fight inflammation. Particular attention to cooking, no frying, but only boiling or grilling. To be preferred, then, are the vegetable proteins of legumes, as they are foods full of fiber and other useful anti-inflammatory substances. Complex carbohydrates, such as whole grains, rice, quinoa, spelled, barley, and millet with wheat, can relieve inflammation, as can the use of certain herbs and spices which, in addition to their antioxidant function, add some flavor in more. In addition to nutrition, it is of fundamental importance to always stay hydrated, especially in the summer season, so a precious piece of advice is to drink plenty of water and, if desired, a cube of at least 80% dark chocolate can be consumed from time to time, always. respecting the portions and without exaggerating.

FOODS TO AVOID:

Let's move on to which foods are not recommended if you decide to follow an anti-inflammatory diet.

 We can assert with absolute certainty that any type of processed, fried, and sweet food is not a wise choice for those who want to reduce inflammation and purify their body. Experts recommend eliminating red meat, chips, alcoholic beverages from your diet. Unfortunately, even desserts do not play in our favor at all, on the other hand, most foods full of sugars do not have the nutrients necessary for our well-being, and being tasty it is very easy to eat more than they should, which would only lead to an increase in weight and, as if that weren't enough, would only increase blood sugar and cholesterol levels, all symptoms that can be related to inflammation. Fizzy drinks, being filled with dyes, preservatives, and additives, can be just as guilty, and many anti-inflammatory diet experts suggest cutting out any foods that may contain added sugar. No refined carbohydrates, i.e. white bread, white pasta, or any product made from white flour. Pre-packaged snacks like crackers and potato chips are to be banished from your cupboard. Finally, we should at least limit the intake of pro-inflammatory foods and animal proteins such as meat, fish, eggs, milk, and cheeses. The problem here is with saturated fats, which can cause inflammation if consumed in excessive doses, this is especially true for processed meats such as sausages, and canned meat.

Example of a typical menu

Here is an example of an anti-inflammatory diet menu. As always, it is recommended that you follow a doctor's dietary directions first.

- **Breakfast**

  o a juice or green tea, coffee to avoid, but if you really can't do without it, drink it in moderation,
  o 100g of seasonal fruit of your choice along with a cup of whole grains,
  o centrifuged fresh fruit and vegetables.

- **Lunch**

  o 60g of pasta or brown rice, or whole grains such as spelled, rye and oats together with legumes and with vegetables garnished with a little extra-virgin olive oil, or tuna salad, a source of omega 3
  o Greek yogurt or a fruit that is low in sugar.

- **Snack**

  o For the snack we can choose between the following alternatives:
  o A handful of dried fruit,
  o 100g of fruit, possibly in season,
  o 125g of low-fat yogurt,
  o Dark chocolate, without exaggerating.

- **Dinner**

  o 150g of grilled or boiled fish, alternatively 120g of turkey or chicken, with vegetables at will, always with a little oil. Avoid red meats,
  o Seasonal fruit or two small squares of dark chocolate, preferably at least 80%, if we feel peckish after dinner.

- As already mentioned, it is recommended to drink a lot of water, regardless of the type of diet.

Should you try it?

Tips to reduce inflammation: Once you have organized the anti-inflammatory diet menu, the ideal would be to try to adopt some good habits and make them fully fit into your daily routine. First of all, regular physical activity is recommended as always, as exercise can reduce inflammatory markers and the risk of chronic diseases. The importance of sleep for our health should not be underestimated, sleeping about eight hours a night, is essential if you do not want to stress your body too much, plus not getting enough rest increases the risk of inflammation. Furthermore, the use of certain supplements can significantly reduce inflammation, but be careful, make sure you need them before taking them. If you combine a healthy lifestyle with a balanced diet, the benefits will be manifold, including an improvement in the symptoms of inflammatory bowel disease and other autoimmune diseases, not to mention a radical decrease in the risk of obesity, heart disease, and diabetes. Following an anti-inflammatory diet could also help reduce certain markers of inflammation in the blood. In addition to this, there will be a marked improvement in glucose levels and a significant increase in energy and good mood.

Anti-Inflammatory Diet Grocery List:

AIP Baking Goods:

Cassava Flour

Arrowroot Flour

Tiger nut Flour

Baking Soda

Carob Powder

Coconut Flour

Coconut Flakes

Banana Flour

Plantain Flour

Sweet Potato Flour

Tapioca Flour

AIP Sweeteners:

Coconut Nectar

Coconut Sugar

Date Sugar

AIP Oils:

Extra Virgin Olive Oil

Coconut Oil

Avocado Oil

AIP Milk:

Coconut Milk

AIP Savory Snacks:

Cassava Bread

Freeze Dried Sweet Potatoes

Jicama Chips

Sweet Potato Chips

Protein Meat Bars

Plantain Strips

Cassava Strips

Meat

Skinless Sardines

Boneless Skinless Salmon

Low Mercury Tuna Cans

Low Mercury Tuna Pouches

AIP Bone Broth:

Organic Chicken Bone Broth

Organic Beef Bone Broth

AIP Condiments:

Nomato Sauce

Coconut Aminos

AIP Seasoning Mix:

AIP Barbecue Sauce

Himalayan Salt

Non Fortified Nutritional Yeast

AIP Noodles:

Sweet Potato Noodles

Kelp Noodles

AIP Sweet Treats:

Coconut Wraps

Power Balls

AIP Supplements:

Powdered Collagen

Powdered Gelatin

... Fruits and Vegetables mentioned in Foods to eat.

MAIN COURSE

(by Chef Amina Subramani)

Honey Garlic Chicken

Ingredients:

1. 1 lb boneless, skinless chicken breasts
2. Salt and black pepper, to taste
3. 2 clove Garlic, minced
4. 1/4 cup flour
5. 2 tablespoon olive oil
6. 2 tablespoon green onions, sliced

Honey Garlic Sauce:

1. 1/2 cup raw honey
2. 3 tablespoon low sodium soy sauce
3. 2 tablespoon olive oil
4. 1 tablespoon hoisin sauce

Instructions:

1. Whisk together honey, light soy sauce, olive oil, and hoisin sauce in a small bowl. Set aside for later.
2. Cut boneless, skinless chicken breasts into pieces. Sprinkle with salt, black pepper and half of the minced garlic. Put the chicken pieces in a mixing bowl. Add the flour, and combine the chicken to coat it evenly with flour.
3. Heat olive oil over medium-high heat. Add the flour coated chicken. Cook for about three minutes, flip the pieces over and cook for another three minutes.
4. Add the remaining garlic, stir and cook for two minutes. Turn the heat down to medium. Add the honey garlic sauce. Stir and cook for 3-4 minutes.
5. Sprinkle with sliced green onions.

Nutrition Calories: 254kcal | Carbohydrates: 21.5g | Protein: 30g | Fat: 6g | Saturated Fat: 1g | Sodium: 294mg| Fiber: 5g

Shepherd's Pie

1. 1 recipe trilogy puree
2. 1 tablespoon ghee
3. 1 ½ lb ground beef
4. Sea salt and pepper
5. 1 cup carrots, diced
6. 1 ½ cup Brussels sprouts, chopped
7. 1 medium onion, chopped
8. 2 cloves garlic, minced
9. 3/4 cup beef bone broth
10. 2 ½ tablespoon tomato paste
11. 1 teaspoon thyme, minced
12. 1 teaspoon rosemary, minced
13. Fresh parsley, chopped, for garnish

Instructions:

1. Heat a pot with water, sprinkle with salt and bring to a boil. Add potato pieces to the boiling water, and cook until very soft.
2. Drain the potatoes and return to the pot. Make heat to low and add the ghee and coconut milk. Mash with a potato masher over very low heat, once smooth, turn heat off and add nutritional yeast, salt and pepper.
3. Preheat your oven to 375 degrees. In a deep oven proof skillet, add beef and sprinkle with sea salt. Brown beef over med-high heat. Remove from skillet to a plate and set aside.
4. Adjust heat to medium and add Brussels sprouts and carrots to skillet, stir to coat and cook about 2 minutes, then add onions and cook until softened. Add garlic and sprinkle veggies with a bit of sea salt, stir, then cover the skillet briefly to soften carrots until fork tender, if necessary.
5. Add the remaining ingredients for the beef mixture to the skillet, stir to combine, then return beef to skillet and stir to coat, simmer for 2 minutes.

6. Spread the trilogy puree over the beef mixture and use a spoon or spatula to smooth the top. Sprinkle with parsley, then place skillet on a large baking sheet and bake in the preheated oven for about 20 minutes, until sauce is bubbling and top begins to turn light brown.
7. Remove from oven, allow to sit about 10 minutes before serving hot. Enjoy!

Nutrition Calories: 383kcal | Carbohydrates: 43g | Protein: 14g | Fat: 19g | Saturated Fat: 3g | Sodium: 1087mg| Fiber: 6.2g

Broccoli Burger recipe

Ingredients:

1. 2½ cups broccoli florets, drained and chopped
2. ¼ cup cassava flour
3. ¼ teaspoon garlic powder
4. 1 tablespoon kosher salt
5. ¼ teaspoon ground black pepper
6. 1 teaspoon vegetable oil
7. 6 AIP hamburger buns, homemade or store bought
8. 6 leaves of lettuce
9. 3 slices white onion, separated into rings
10. Tomato, sliced

Instructions:

1. Bring 2 quarts of water and ½ tablespoon of salt to a boil in a large pot. Boil broccoli for 3 minutes and transfer to a bowl of ice water. Drain broccoli and squeeze out the extra moisture.
2. Rough chop broccoli and place into a medium bowl with flour, garlic powder, ½ teaspoon kosher salt, black pepper. Mix ingredients thoroughly until mixture binds and becomes shapeable. Divide mixture into 6 even portions and form each portion into a patty.
3. Preheat a large skillet with vegetable oil on medium heat for 2 minutes. Reduce heat to med-low heat and add broccoli patties to the pan. Cook for 2 minutes on each side.
4. To assemble, place the patty on top, then the lettuce, onion, tomato, and the top bun last. Enjoy and serve with ketchup if desired. You can use vegan mayonnaise if you have a taste for it.

Nutrition Calories: 152kcal | Carbohydrates: 26g | Protein: 6g | Fat: 3g | Saturated Fat: 0.4g | Sodium: 217mg| Fiber: 4.6g

Mexican Ground Beef Skillet

1. 1 lb ground beef
2. 2 medium sweet potatoes, diced
3. 1 medium red onion, finely diced
4. 2 stalks kale, chopped
5. 2 teaspoon dried oregano
6. 2 teaspoon garlic powder
7. 2 teaspoon onion powder
8. Salt, to taste
9. Juice of one lime
10. For garnish: Avocado, Cilantro, Fresh salsa

Instructions:

1. Heat the stove on medium and prepare a large skillet. Add the ground beef to the pan and lightly salt. Cook on medium heat until browned, and set aside.
2. Add the sweet potatoes and cook until softened and crisped, stirring frequently, Add in the red onion and cook until the onions are translucent.
3. Add the kale and cook for 2-3 minutes or until wilted. Add back in the beef, along with the salt, pepper, cumin, oregano, onion powder, garlic, lime juice and stir for until well combined.
4. To serve, top with avocado, cilantro, and salsa.

Nutrition Calories: 192kcal | Carbohydrates: 18g | Protein: 5.2g | Fat: 12g | Saturated Fat: 7g | Sodium: 1034mg| Fiber: 4.7g

Sweet Potato Avocado Toast

Ingredients

1. 1 large sweet potato
2. 1 large Avocado
3. ½ cup tomato, lightly sliced
4. Salt and pepper, to taste
5. 3 clove garlic, minced

Instructions:

1. Using a large sharp knife, slice the sweet potato lengthwise down the middle, make 1/4"-1/3" thick from the middle of the sweet potato.
2. Place slices in a toaster on high for about 5 minutes or until cooked through. Meanwhile, mash the avocado in a bowl. Add sliced tomatoes and minced garlic. Stir to combine.
3. Top the sweet potato toast with avocado mixture.

Nutrition Calories: 489kcal | Carbohydrates: 65g | Protein: 10g | Fat: 21g | Saturated Fat: 3g | Sodium: 503mg| Fiber: 5g

Shrimp Scampi with Zucchini Noodles

Ingredients:

1. 3 tablespoon olive oil
2. 3 cloves garlic, minced
3. 1 lb shrimp, peeled deveined
4. Juice of 1 lemon
5. 1 teaspoon lemon zest
6. 1/4 cup chicken broth
7. 3 tablespoon ghee
8. 3 tablespoon parsley, chopped
9. Salt and pepper, to taste
10. 2 large zucchini

Instructions:

1. Combine 1 tablespoon oil and 1 clove garlic. Brush over the shrimp and let marinate for 30 minutes.
2. Heat remaining 2 tablespoon oil in a large sauce pan. Add shrimp and cook for 1-2 minutes per side, Set aside.
3. Keeping oil on the pan, Add remaining garlic and saute for 1 minute, until fragrant. Put in lemon juice, chicken broth, and zest. Cook for another 3 minutes until sauce is reduced.
4. Add ghee to the pan. Continue to cook for another 3 minutes until sauce begins to thicken. Add shrimp back to the pan and cook for another 2 minutes per side, coating with the sauce along the way.
5. To make the zucchini noodles, spiralize the zucchini. Add about 1 tablespoon oil, and saute for 5 minutes. Toss shrimp and sauce with zucchini.
6. Top with fresh parsley to serve.

Nutrition Calories: 435kcal | Carbohydrates: 5g | Protein: 32g | Fat: 31g | Saturated Fat: 11g | Sodium: 1259mg| Fiber: 1g

Lettuce Burger recipe

Ingredients:

1. 1 lb ground beef
2. 2 tablespoon ghee
3. Salt and pepper
4. 1 onion, sliced into rings
5. 1 tomato, sliced
6. 1 dill pickle, sliced into rounds
7. 1 head iceberg lettuce

For the sauce:

1. 2 tablespoon tomato paste
2. 1 tablespoon white vinegar
3. 1 teaspoon mustard
4. 1 teaspoon coconut aminos
5. 1/4 teaspoon garlic powder
6. 1/4 teaspoon onion powder
7. 1/4 cup mayo
8. 1 small dill pickle, finely diced

Instructions:

1. To prepare the sauce, Combine all of the sauce ingredients in a bowl and mix well with a whisk. Refrigerate while you make the burgers.
2. Form beef into burger patties. Season the patties with salt and pepper on both sides and set aside.
3. Heat a skillet over medium-low heat and add 1 tablespoon of ghee. Add the onion to cook, stirring occasionally, until browned.
4. Cook over medium-high heat on a grill or heat a large skillet over medium-high heat and add 1 tablespoon ghee. Once the

ghee is hot, add the burgers to cook for 3-4 minutes per side, or until cooked.

5. Put 1/2 of the lettuce wedge on a plate and add a tomato slice and some pickles at the bottom. Top with a burger patty and spread some sauce over the top.

6. Add on some onions and top with more sauce if desired. Top with the other 1/2 of the lettuce wedge to form a burger. Pick it up with both hands and enjoy!

Nutrition Calories: 498kcal | Carbohydrates: 10g | Protein: 22g | Fat: 41g | Saturated Fat: 15g | Sodium: 197mg| Fiber: 3g

Healthy Baked Salmon

Ingredients:

1. 4 salmon fillets
2. 2 tablespoons olive oil
3. Salt and cracked pepper, to taste
4. 2 teaspoons garlic, minced
5. 1/4 teaspoon each dried thyme, parsley, oregano, and basil
6. 1 medium lemon

Instructions:

1. Preheat oven to 400 degrees and grease a large baking pan. Arrange salmon fillets on the baking sheet and season generously with salt and pepper.
2. Stir together olive oil, garlic, herbs, and juice of 1/2 lemon. Spoon over salmon fillets being sure to rub all over the tops and sides of the salmon.
3. Thinly slice remaining 1/2 of lemon and top each piece of salmon with a slice of lemon.
4. Bake for 15-18 minutes until salmon is opaque and flaky when pulled apart. Garnish with fresh thyme or parsley if desired and serve.

Nutrition Calories: 355kcal | Carbohydrates: 30g | Protein: 26g | Fat: 14g | Saturated Fat: 3g | Sodium: 185mg| Fiber: 2.5g

Roasted Cauliflower Soup

Ingredients:

1. 1 large head cauliflower, cut into florets
2. 2 tablespoon olive oil
3. 1 tablespoon coconut oil
4. 1 medium white onion, chopped
5. 2 cloves garlic, minced
6. 3 cups homemade vegetable broth
7. 2 tablespoon nutritional yeast
8. 1 tablespoon lemon juice

Instructions:

1. Preheat oven to 425F. On a baking sheet, toss cauliflower with olive oil and sprinkle with salt. Bake until browned, about 25 minutes.
2. Add the coconut oil in an oven over medium heat. Once melted add onion and cook until translucent. Add the garlic and stir until fragrant.
3. Add the broth and cauliflower to the pot. Cook for 10 minutes and then transfer carefully to a blender.
4. Add the nutritional yeast, and lemon juice to the blender. Blend until smooth. Serve and enjoy!

Nutrition Calories: 129kcal | Carbohydrates: 28g | Protein: 5g | Fat: 0.2g | Saturated Fat: 0.1g | Sodium: 953mg| Fiber: 6.8g

Stuffed Mushroom

Ingredients:

1. 40 large white mushrooms
2. ¼ cup roasted red bell pepper, chopped
3. ½ medium onion
4. 3 green onions
5. 1 teaspoon oregano
6. 6 tablespoon (cassava flour) breadcrumbs
7. ¼ cup parsley fresh
8. 2 tablespoon olive oil
9. Salt, to taste

Instructions:

1. Preheat oven to 400 F degrees. Place the mushrooms stem side down on a baking sheet and bake until the liquid leaks out of them.
2. Chop up about half the mushroom stems in very small pieces. Chop the onion, green onions, red bell pepper, roasted pepper and parsley.
3. Heat 2 tablespoon of olive oil in a skillet. Add the mushrooms stems, red pepper, roasted pepper, green onion and onion to the skillet and saute. Add the oregano and salt and pepper. Saute for about 5 minutes until pepper and onion are tender.
4. Transfer the stuffing to a bowl and let it cool a bit. Add the parsley and breadcrumbs and mix well.
5. Place the mushrooms stem side up on the baking sheet and fill them with the stuffing, generously. Bake for 15 minutes. Serve warm.

Nutrition Calories: 85kcal | Carbohydrates: 9g | Protein: 4g | Fat: 4g | Saturated Fat: 1.7g | Sodium: 246mg| Fiber: 1g

Harvest Bowl

Ingredients:

For the bowl:

1. 1 tablespoon avocado/coconut oil
2. 1 lb boneless, skinless Chicken Thighs
3. 3 Sweet Potatoes
4. 1 teaspoon Sea Salt
5. ¼ teaspoon Cinnamon
6. 4 cups Baby Spinach
7. 2 Green Apples, diced
8. ¼ cup Raisins

For the sauce:

1. 2 tablespoon Apple Cider Vinegar
2. ¼ cup Olive Oil
3. Salt, to taste

Instructions:

1. Preheat the oven to 425 F. Line baking sheets with parchment paper. Peel and dice the sweet potatoes into 1/2-inch pieces for diced potatoes. Toss with the ½ teaspoon salt, cinnamon, and 1 tablespoon oil and then place on the baking sheet.
2. Season the chicken with the remaining 1/2 teaspoon salt and then place on the other sheet pan. Place both the sweet potatoes and chicken in the oven and roast for 30-35 minutes.
3. Meanwhile, make the sauce by whisking all of the sauce ingredients together. Once the sweet potatoes and chicken are done, divide the ingredients between the bowls, add some raisins, drizzle the sauce and serve.

Nutrition Calories: 270kcal | Carbohydrates: 19g | Protein: 15g | Fat: 13g | Saturated Fat: 4g | Sodium: 1530mg| Fiber: 1g

Squash Pasta Salad

Ingredients:

For the salad:

1. 2 ½ lb yellow squash, peeled and spiralized into noodles
2. ½ cup green onions, sliced
3. ½ large cucumber, sliced
4. 1 (6 oz) can black olives, halved

For the dressing:

1. ½ cup olive oil
2. 3 tablespoon apple cider vinegar
3. ½ teaspoon garlic powder
4. ¾ teaspoon onion powder
5. 1 teaspoon oregano
6. ¼ teaspoon black pepper
7. 1 teaspoon of thyme and basil
8. Fresh Parsley, chopped
9. Salt, to taste

Instructions:

1. Place all veggies in a large bowl. Place all dressing ingredients in a small other bowl. Shake in mix thoroughly.
2. Pour dressing over veggies and toss to combine. Serve cold.

Nutrition Calories: 225kcal | Carbohydrates: 36.7g | Protein: 7g | Fat: 6g | Saturated Fat: 0.8g | Sodium: 145mg| Fiber: 2.7g

Teriyaki Meatballs

Ingredients:

For the meatballs:

1. 2 pound chicken
2. 6 cloves garlic, minced
3. 1 teaspoon ginger, minced
4. 1 teaspoon coconut aminos
5. 1 teaspoon onion powder
6. ½ teaspoon red pepper flakes

For the teriyaki sauce:

1. ¾ cup coconut aminos
2. 2 tablespoon lime juice
3. 3 cloves garlic
4. 1 teaspoon ginger
5. 1 tablespoon avocado oil
6. 2 tablespoon water+ 2 teaspoon arrowroot flour

Instructions:

1. Preheat the oven to 400. Put a non-stick baking pan.
2. Mix the meatball mixture in a large mixing bowl. Now, use a 1 inch cookie scoop and scoop the meatballs out. You should be able to make roughly 22. Now bake the meatballs for 25 minutes.
3. Meanwhile, add all of the sauce ingredients in a saucepan on medium heat except the arrowroot and water. Bring to a boil.
4. In a separate bowl, add the water and arrowroot and whisk together. Now, add the arrowroot mixture to the saucepan and whisk together for 1 minute until the sauce thickens.
5. Once it thickens, add the sauce and the meatballs into a clean bowl and toss and enjoy!

Nutrition Calories: 185kcal | Carbohydrates: 6.7g | Protein: 17g | Fat: 10g | Saturated Fat: 4g | Sodium: 382mg| Fiber: 0.1g

Beef Lettuce Wrap

Ingredients:

1. 2 tablespoons olive oil
2. 1 medium onion, sliced
3. 1 lb beef
4. 2 cup beef broth
5. 2 teaspoons coconut aminos
6. 2 teaspoons honey
7. Iceberg lettuce, to serve
8. Fresh parsley, to garnish

Instructions:

1. In a pan, cook onions with one tablespoon olive oil until soft and caramelized. Remove and set aside.
2. In the same pan, heat the second tablespoon olive oil and brown the beef on all sides until golden and caramelized. Transfer the beef to the crockpot and add the cooked onions and hot beef stock. Cover and cook for 5 hours.3
3. Remove the beef and place into a bowl. Cover with foil and allow to rest. Pour the leftover juices in the crockpot into a clean pan on the stove and reduce over moderate heat. Stir in the coconut aminos and honey, and reduce the heat to low.
4. Once the beef has rested for 10 minutes, shred into pieces and place back in bowl. Pour the sauce over the meat and stir well to combine.
5. Spoon the beef into lettuce cups and garnish with parsley.

Nutrition Calories: 267kcal | Carbohydrates: 16g | Protein: 21g | Fat: 12g | Saturated Fat: 4g | Sodium: 677mg| Fiber: 3g

Shrimp and Asparagus

Ingredients:

1. 3 tablespoon avocado oil
2. 8 oz asparagus
3. 3 clove garlic, minced
4. ½ cup cilantro, chopped
5. 1 pound medium shrimp, deveined and shell removed
6. Salt, to taste

Instructions:

1. Snap off the ends of the asparagus stalks and cut into 2" pieces or whole if you wish
2. Heat the avocado oil in a large skillet. When the oil is shimmering, Add shrimp, minced garlic and a pinch of salt and allow to cook for about 2-3 minutes.
3. Add asparagus and cook until shrimp are uniformly pink and cooked through, stirring frequently, about 3-4 minutes.
4. Remove from heat and stir in the cilantro. Serve and enjoy!

Nutrition Calories: 384kcal | Carbohydrates: 54g | Protein: 21g | Fat: 11g | Saturated Fat: 1g | Sodium: 734mg| Fiber: 8g

Chicken Burritos

Ingredients:

1. 1 pound chicken, chopped or shredded
2. 3/4 pound bacon, chopped
3. 1 small onion, chopped
4. 1 teaspoon ground ginger
5. ¼ teaspoon garlic powder
6. ¼ teaspoon dried oregano
7. 1 cup guacamole or salsa, optional
8. Avocado slices, to top
9. 6 cassava flour tortillas, homemade or store bought

Instructions:

1. Combine the meat, bacon, tomato sauce, onion, ginger, garlic powder, and oregano in a slow cooker and cook on high for 2 hours. Meanwhile, make the tortillas.
2. Shred the meat and scoop it into the tortillas, then top with guacamole, avocado or other toppings.

Nutrition Calories: 698kcal | Carbohydrates: 38g | Protein: 46g | Fat: 41g | Saturated Fat: 11g | Sodium: 1756mg| Fiber: 6g

Chicken Quesadillas

Ingredients:

1. 1 tablespoon Ghee
2. 1 Yellow Onion
3. 8 Grain-Free Tortillas, any variety
4. 2-3 Pan-Fried Chicken Tenders
5. Salsa or Tomatoes, to serve
6. Fresh Chives, to serve, optional

Instructions:

1. Halve and thinly slice the onions. Melt 1 tablespoon of ghee in a skillet over medium-high heat and add the onions. Saute, stirring occasionally, until onions are translucent, browned, and fragrant. Remove onions from skillet and set aside.
2. Wipe out the skillet so it's ready for the tortillas. Chop the chicken tenders into small, bite-size pieces. Set aside.
3. Place the skillet over medium heat and let it heat up while you prepare the tortillas. Spread a very thin layer of ghee on one side of ghee each tortilla. Place one tortilla, ghee side down, on the warm skillet.
4. Spread on some sauted onions, and sprinkle on some of the chopped chicken pieces. Top with another tortilla, ghee side up. Let cook, undisturbed, in the skillet for about 3 minutes, or until the bottom tortilla is crispy and browned.
5. Using a large spatula, flip the quesadilla and cook the other side for an additional 2 minutes or so, until browned. Remove from skillet and cut into 4 triangles. Serve hot with diced tomatoes and chopped chives.

Nutrition Calories: 273kcal | Carbohydrates: 28g | Protein: 13g | Fat: 12g | Saturated Fat: 6g | Sodium: 525mg| Fiber: 3g

Vegetarian chow mein

1. 2 (3 oz) of any grain-free noodles
2. 2 tablespoons olive oil
3. 1 medium carrot, peeled and cut into slices
4. 3.5oz broccoli florets, chopped
5. 2 clove garlic cloves, minced
6. 1/2 thumb-size piece (3 g) fresh ginger, minced
7. 2 tablespoons coconut aminos
8. 2 teaspoons honey

Instructions:

1. Rinse the noodles under cold water and place into a pan of warm, simmering water. Set aside to warm noodles while you make the stir-fry.
2. Heat the olive oil over medium heat and fry the carrots and broccoli until slightly softened. Add the garlic and ginger, and fry for an additional 2-3 minutes, stirring regularly.
3. Pour in the coconut aminos and honey and increase the heat toward until the sauce reduces and coats the vegetables.
4. Drain the noodles and add the vegetable stir fry. Combine together and serve.

Nutrition Calories: 317kcal | Carbohydrates: 48g | Protein: 12g | Fat: 10g | Saturated Fat: 2g | Sodium: 780mg| Fiber: 4g

Broccoli Chicken Casserole

Ingredients

1. 3 cups roasted spaghetti squash
2. 2 cups raw broccoli florets, small pieces
3. 2 cups shredded chicken
4. 2 tablespoons coconut oil
5. 2 tablespoons arrowroot flour
6. 1 cup bone broth
7. 1 cup coconut milk
8. 1 ½ teaspoon salt
9. ½ tablespoon nutritional yeast
10. 1 cup pork panko

Instructions:

1. Preheat the oven to 350 degrees F. Spread spaghetti squash evenly on the bottom of a baking dish. Spread broccoli evenly over the squash. Spread the chicken evenly over all. Set aside.
2. In a saucepan over medium high heat, melt coconut oil. Add arrowroot flour, and whisk until smooth. Whisk in the broth and coconut milk. Turn heat to high. Whisk constantly while it bubbles and thickens.
3. When it has thickened to the consistency of gravy, turn heat back down to medium high. Whisk in the salt and nutritional yeast. Pour the sauce evenly over the vegetables and chicken. Sprinkle it all with pork panko.
4. Bake uncovered for 30 minutes. Let it sit for a bit before serving, about five minutes. Makes great leftovers!

Nutrition Calories: 429kcal | Carbohydrates: 7g | Protein: 32g | Fat: 30g | Saturated Fat: 11g | Sodium: 670mg| Fiber: 0g

Chicken with vegetable Curry

Ingredients:

1. 1 (15-ounce) can full fat coconut milk
2. 2 tablespoon ginger, minced
3. 3 cloves garlic, minced
4. 2 large carrots, sliced
5. 1 large crown broccoli, chopped into florets
6. 1 yellow squash, chopped
7. 1 large boneless skinless chicken breast
8. 2 tablespoon coconut aminos
9. 1 teaspoon ground turmeric
10. ½ teaspoon ground cinnamon
11. Salt, to taste
12. ¼ cup fresh basil, chopped

Instructions:

1. Pour 1/4 cup of the coconut milk into a large skillet and heat to medium. Add the ginger and garlic, and cook until fragrant, about 2 to 3 minutes.
2. Add the carrots and broccoli and cover. Cook, stirring occasionally, until veggies have softened but are still al dente, about 3 minutes.
3. Heat a small amount of coconut oil in a separate skillet over medium heat. Add the chopped chicken. Brown the chicken, stirring occasionally, about 5 minutes.
4. Strain the liquid from the chicken, then add the chicken to the skillet with the vegetables.
5. Add all the remaining ingredients including the remaining coconut milk except for the basil to the skillet with the vegetables and chicken. Stir well and bring to a full boil, then reduce the heat to a simmer and cover.
6. Cook 15 minutes, then uncover and continue cooking another 8 to 10 minutes, until curry has thickened and chicken is cooked through. Garnish with basil.

Nutrition Calories: 371kcal | Carbohydrates: 47g | Protein: 8g | Fat: 20g | Saturated Fat: 8g | Sodium: 256mg| Fiber: 10g

Spinach Chicken herb Soup

Ingredients

1. 1 lb ground chicken
2. 2 teaspoon garlic, minced
3. ½ teaspoon lemon zest
4. ¼ cup fresh parsley, chopped
5. 1 teaspoon dried basil
6. 2 teaspoon Salt
7. 2 teaspoon extra-virgin olive oil
8. 1 cup onion, finely chopped
9. ½ cup celery, finely chopped
10. ½ cup carrot, grated
11. 1 cup bone broth
12. 4 cup baby spinach
13. ¼ cup dill, chopped
14. 2 tablespoon lemon juice

Instructions:

1. Preheat oven to 350 degrees. In a large bowl, combine the first five ingredients plus one teaspoon of salt.
2. With a teaspoon, scoop out the prepared mixture onto a parchment lined roasting sheet by forming a shape of ball. Bake meatballs for 30 minutes.
3. Meanwhile, Heat olive oil in a soup pot over medium high heat. Add onions, celery, and carrots. Saute for 5 minutes. Add bone broth, meatballs, dill, and one teaspoon of salt. Bring to a full simmer.
4. Add spinach and simmer for about a minute. Stir in lemon juice. Serve and enjoy.

Nutrition Calories: 296kcal | Carbohydrates: 15g | Protein: 40g | Fat: 9g | Saturated Fat: 4g | Sodium: 20mg| Fiber: 5g

Cauliflower Risotto

Ingredients:

1. 1 tablespoon extra-virgin olive oil
2. 1 yellow onion, diced
3. 8 ounces mushrooms, sliced (any variety)
4. 12 ounces asparagus , cut into 1" pieces
5. 1 clove garlic, minced
6. 1 tablespoon balsamic vinegar
7. ½ teaspoon dried thyme
8. 1 pound cauliflower rice (homemade or store bought)
9. ¾ cup coconut milk
10. Salt, to taste

Instructions:

1. Prepare the cauliflower rice if you haven't bought them. Heat the olive oil in a large skillet over medium heat. Saute the onion until it starts to soften, about 5 minutes, then add in the mushrooms and asparagus and cook for 5 more minutes.
2. Add in the garlic, balsamic vinegar, and thyme and saute for another minute. Add in the prepared cauliflower rice, coconut milk, and 1 teaspoon of salt, then stir well.
3. Bring the coconut milk to a simmer and cover the pot with a lid. Lower the heat and let the vegetables cook until the cauliflower rice is tender, about 10 minutes.
4. Serve warm with green onions on top.

Nutrition Calories: 156kcal | Carbohydrates: 9g | Protein: 6g | Fat: 9g | Saturated Fat: 3g | Sodium: 1173mg| Fiber: 7g

Cassava flour Naan Flatbread

Ingredients:

1. 1 ¼ cup cassava flour
2. ½ teaspoon baking soda
3. Salt, to taste
4. 2 tablespoon avocado or olive oil
5. ¼ cup Non-dairy milk
6. 1 teaspoon apple cider vinegar
7. Avocado or coconut oil, for cooking

Instructions:

1. In a bowl, sift the flour, baking soda and some salt. Combine well using your hand or a spoon. Next slowly mix in the milk, 2 tablespoon oil, and a mix together.
2. Next slowly add water little at a time until you get a pizza dough like texture. Roll the dough into 4 -6 medium size balls. Place dough balls on a clean space and roll each one until you form an oval shape. Shape the corners to round after.
3. Heat a non-stick pan with oil on medium high. Place each flattened dough on pan one at a time on medium high heat. Cover with lid and wait for few seconds. You will start to see the edges puff up.
4. Drizzle a splash of more oil on top and flip to other side. Cover and cook an additional 1-2 minutes. Remove and repeat for the next until you get 4-6 naan breads.
5. Serve with your favorite side dishes.

Nutrition Calories: 250kcal | Carbohydrates: 45g | Protein: 9g | Fat: 3g | Saturated Fat: 0.4g | Sodium: 390mg| Fiber: 2g

Healthy Burrito bowl

1. 1 pound skinless, boneless chicken thighs
2. 3 tablespoons avocado oil
3. 2 cups cauliflower rice, frozen
4. ½ onion, sliced
5. 1 radish, quartered
6. Salt, to taste
7. 1 teaspoon ginger, minced
8. 1 teaspoon parsley
9. 1 teaspoon ground turmeric
10. Romaine lettuce and chopped avocados, to serve

For the Dressing:

1. ½ cup cilantro, stems trimmed
2. 2 tablespoon lemon juice
3. 1 tablespoon apple cider vinegar
4. 2 tablespoons coconut butter
5. 1 tablespoon nutritional yeast
6. 1 tablespoon coconut aminos
7. ½ cup avocado oil and salt, to taste

Instructions:

1. Preheat the oven to 400F. Drizzle one tablespoon of avocado oil all over a sheet pan. One on side spread out 2 cups of frozen cauliflower rice.
2. Next to it, line up the chicken in a single layer. In the space that is left arrange the red onion and radishes. Sprinkle the salt over everything, getting about 1 teaspoon on the chicken thighs.
3. Add the remaining seasoning only to the chicken. Then drizzle the rest of the oil all over the chicken and rice. Put the sheet

pan in the oven and roast for 30 minutes. Then broil for 5 minutes.

4. Meanwhile, make the sauce. Combine the cilantro, nutritional yeast, lemon juice, coconut butter, salt and coconut aminos in the blender, and blend on low until almost smooth. Then slowly drizzle in the avocado oil until the sauce is fluid. Set aside.

5. To assemble your bowls make a bed of romaine in two bowls. Then spoon the rice on one side, the radishes onions and avocado on another. Slice 2 chicken thighs per bowl. Then drizzle sauce over everything. There will be extra sauce. Store it in the fridge and use as salad dressing!

Nutrition Calories: 356kcal | Carbohydrates: 20g | Protein: 19g | Fat: 21g | Saturated Fat: 8g | Sodium: 617mg| Fiber: 2.5g

Zucchini Lasagna

Ingredients:

1. 1 pound white-fleshed sweet potato, peeled
2. 2 cups zucchini, shredded
3. 2 cups yellow squash, shredded
4. 4 tablespoons avocado oil
5. 1 lb ground turkey
6. 1 tablespoon fresh thyme, chopped
7. 1 tablespoon fresh oregano, chopped
8. 6 cloves garlic, minced
9. Salt, to taste

Instructions:

1. Preheat oven to 375 and grease a pan. Take your peeled white yams, and slice them lengthwise to 1/8" thickness. Set noodles aside.
2. In a large skillet, heat 2 tablespoons of the avocado oil over medium-high heat. Add turkey and half a teaspoon of the salt and brown for 7-9 minutes, until cooked through. Stir occasionally.
3. Meanwhile, shred zucchini and squash in a food processor using the shredder attachment. Remove turkey from the pan and set aside.
4. Add squash, zucchini, thyme, garlic and oregano to the hot pan. Season with 1/2 teaspoon sea salt and saute for 5 minutes. Remove skillet from heat and set aside.
5. Layer 1/3 of the sweet potato noodles on the bottom of the pan. Brush noodles with 1/3 of the remaining oil. Top with half of the zucchini mixture, then half of the meat mixture. Repeat once, and end with the noodles.

6. Brush top layer of noodles with the last third of the oil mixture. Season with salt to taste. Cover lasagna with foil and bake for 35 minutes. Uncover, raise oven temp to 450, and bake an additional 15 minutes, until the top is golden brown. Allow to cool for at least 10 minutes before serving.

Nutrition Calories: 270kcal | Carbohydrates: 18g | Protein: 11g | Fat: 17g | Saturated Fat: 2g | Sodium: 150mg| Fiber: 1g

Beef Bourguignon

Ingredients

1. 1 tablespoons extra-virgin olive oil
2. 6 ounces (170g) bacon, chopped
3. 3 pounds beef, cut into 2" chunks
4. 1 large carrot, sliced
5. 1 large white onion, diced
6. 6 cloves garlic, minced
7. Salt, to taste
8. 2 tablespoons cassava flour
9. 3 cups red wine
10. 2 cups beef stock
11. 2 tablespoons tomato paste
12. 1 beef cube, crushed
13. 1 teaspoon fresh thyme, chopped
14. 2 tablespoons fresh parsley, chopped
15. 2 bay leaves
16. 1 pound small mushrooms, quartered
17. 2 tablespoons ghee

Instructions:

1. In a large oven, saute the bacon over medium heat in 1 tablespoon of oil for about 3 minutes, until crisp and browned. Transfer with a slotted spoon to a large dish and set aside.
2. Pat dry beef with paper towel; sear in batches in the hot oil until browned on all sides. Remove to the dish with the bacon.
3. In the remaining oil, saute the carrots and diced onions until softened, then add 4 cloves minced garlic and cook for 1 minute. Drain excess fat and return the bacon and beef back into the pot; season with 1/2 teaspoon salt.

4. Sprinkle with flour, toss well and cook for 4-5 minutes to brown. 4. Add the wine and enough stock so that the meat is barely covered. Then add the tomato paste, bullion and herbs. Cover and bring to a boil, then reduce heat to low and simmer for 1 ½ to 2 hours, stirring occasionally, until the meat is falling apart.

5. Prepare your mushrooms, Heat the butter in a medium-sized skillet/pan over heat. When the foam subsides, add the remaining 2 cloves garlic and cook until fragrant, then add in the mushrooms. Cook for about 5 minutes, while shaking the pan occasionally to coat with the butter. Season with salt and pepper, if desired. Once they are browned, set aside.

6. Place a colander over a large pot. Remove the casserole from the oven and carefully empty its contents into the colander. Discard the herbs.

7. Return the beef mixture back into the oven. Add the mushrooms over the meat. Remove any fat off the sauce and simmer for a minute or two, skimming off any additional fat which rises to the surface.

8. Pour the sauce over the meat and vegetables. Simmer the beef bourguignon for 2 to 3 minutes to heat through. Garnish with parsley and serve.

Nutrition Calories: 341kcal | Carbohydrates: 26g | Protein: 31g | Fat: 10g | Saturated Fat: 3g | Sodium: 837mg| Fiber: 10g

Grilled Fish Tacos

Ingredients:

1. 3 fillets cod
2. 1 lime
3. 1/2 teaspoon garlic powder
4. 2 oranges, peeled and diced
5. 1 large carrot, julienne peeled
6. 1 cup green cabbage, thinly sliced
7. 2 tablespoon fresh cilantro, chopped
8. 1 lime juiced Salt, to taste
9. Salt, to taste
10. 6 cassava flour tortillas

Instructions:

1. Combine orange, carrot, cabbage, cilantro and some salt to taste together in a bowl and set aside.
2. Heat a grill on medium-high heat and grill the fish for 2-3 minutes on one side. Squeeze the lime over the fish and season with garlic and salt. Flip the fish and grill for another 2-3 minutes.
3. Assemble the fish tacos by placing small pieces of fish in each taco, then top with the slaw. Garnish with avocado and lime slices if desired.

Nutrition Calories: 517kcal | Carbohydrates: 31g | Protein: 84g | Fat: 5g | Saturated Fat: 1g | Sodium: 459mg| Fiber: 4g

Chicken Alfredo recipe

1. Olive Oil
2. 1 chicken breast, skin on
3. 1 zucchini, spiralized
4. ¾ cup coconut cream
5. 1 tablespoon cassava flour
6. 1 tablespoon coconut oil
7. 1 cup chicken broth
8. 1 tablespoon nutritional yeast
9. 2 clove garlic, minced
10. 4 tablespoons fresh parsley, chopped
11. Salt, to taste

Instructions:

1. Heat a drizzle of oil in a nonstick pan over medium-high heat. Place the chicken breast in the skillet and cook for 5 minutes on each side or until the skin is golden and the chicken is cooked through. Remove the chicken from the skillet and set aside.
2. Melt the coconut oil in the same pan over medium heat. Add the cassava flour to the pan and whisk to create a paste.
3. Slowly add the chicken broth, a little at a time, while continuously whisking to combine. Once all the chicken broth has been incorporated, add the coconut cream and whisk until fully combined.
4. Add the garlic, nutritional yeast, and fresh parsley to the pan and bring to a boil. Reduce the heat to a simmer and continue to cook for about 5 minutes or until thickened, stirring occasionally. Season with salt, to taste.
5. Pour the sauce into a blender or food processor and blend for 30 seconds. Add the zucchini 'noodles' to the pan and saute for

about 2 minutes. Return the sauce to the pan and heat through. Slice the chicken breast and place it on top of the "noodles" and Alfredo sauce. Garnish with optional chopped fresh parsley and serve.

Nutrition Calories: 300kcal | Carbohydrates: 40g | Protein: 20g | Fat: 7g | Saturated Fat: 3g | Sodium: 660mg| Fiber: 4g

Crockpot Chicken Stew

Ingredients:

1. 2 lbs chicken breasts
2. 5 carrots, chopped
3. 1 ½ onion, roughly chopped
4. 2 ½ apples, roughly chopped
5. 10 pitted plums
6. 1 can coconut milk
7. Salt, to taste
8. Fresh Rosemary or thyme, chopped, for garnish

Instructions:

1. Cut up the chicken into chunks and place it in your slow cooker. Add the carrots, the onions and then the apples.
2. Add in 10 plums. Pour the coconut milk all over the ingredients. Cook for 8 hours in your slow cooker.
3. Salt the stew to taste when the crock-pot is almost done, mixing all the ingredients together.
4. Serve with a sprinkle of fresh rosemary or thyme.

Nutrition Calories: 130kcal | Carbohydrates: 13g | Protein: 9g | Fat: 5g | Saturated Fat: 1g | Sodium: 700mg| Fiber: 1g

Cauliflower Fried Rice

1. 6 cups riced cauliflower
2. ½ cup coconut oil
3. 2 cups broccoli, chopped
4. 2 cups carrots, chopped
5. 1 cup green onion, chopped
6. ½ cup coconut aminos
7. 1 teaspoon ground ginger
8. ½ teaspoon ground cumin
9. Salt, to taste
10. ¼ teaspoon turmeric
11. 1 tablespoon honey or maple syrup

Instructions:

1. Place a large pan on the stove on medium heat. Add the coconut oil to the pan and allow it to melt. Add the chopped broccoli, carrots and green onion to the pan. Cook for about 10 minutes.
2. While the vegetables are cooking, mix up the sauce in a glass measuring cup or bowl. Add the riced cauliflower to the pan and stir together with the other vegetables
3. Add the sauce and stir well to combine. Cook for an additional 15-20 minutes. Serve and enjoy with a slice of cucumber.

Nutrition Calories: 191kcal | Carbohydrates: 15g | Protein: 5.7g | Fat: 14g | Saturated Fat: 2g | Sodium: 86.3mg| Fiber: 7.2g

SECOND COURSE

(by Chef Amina Subramani)

Beef Stir Fry

1. 1 lb steak, thinly sliced
2. 1 medium yellow zucchini, sliced
3. 1 medium onion, sliced
4. 1 bell pepper, sliced (any choice of color)
5. 1/2 lb mushrooms, thinly sliced
6. 1 teaspoon ginger, minced
7. 1 clove garlic, minced
8. 3 tablespoon Oil to Saute
9. ¼ cup AIP BBQ Sauce

Instructions:

1. Heat a large heavy pan, add 1 tablespoon oil. When oil become hot, add beef and saute for 2-3 minutes. Stir and saute another 2 minute or until nearly cooked through. Season lightly with salt and pepper, add ginger and garlic and saute.
2. Drizzle beef with AIP sauce to taste, and stir-fry, until beef is fully cooked through. Remove beef to a plate and cover to keep warm.
3. Place clean pan over high heat and add 1 tablespoon oil. Once hot, add mushrooms, season lightly with salt and pepper and stir fry until golden. Transfer mushrooms to the plate with beef.
4. Add remaining tablespoon of oil along with sliced onion and veggies and stir fry about 8 min or until soft and golden. Combine vegetables with beef and mushrooms, drizzle in more sauce to taste and stir fry just until hot. Serve with your favorite dish.

Nutrition Calories: 180kcal | Carbohydrates: 29g | Protein: 11g | Fat: 2g | Saturated Fat: 1g | Sodium: 980mg| Fiber: 4g

Instant Pot Turmeric Chicken

Ingredients:

1. 3 tablespoons olive oil
2. 3 medium red onions, diced
3. 2 bay leaves
4. 8 cloves
5. 1 cinnamon stick
6. 1½ pounds chicken thighs
7. Salt, to taste
8. ½ teaspoon turmeric powder
9. 1 teaspoon garlic, minced
10. 1½ teaspoons ginger, minced
11. 2 medium sweet potatoes, cut into ¼-inch thick
12. Cilantro, for garnish

Instructions:

1. Add extra virgin olive oil, sliced onions, bay leaves, cloves, and cinnamon stick to your instant pot. Let them brown for about 6 minutes over medium heat. Stir often to prevent from burning.
2. Put the chicken and let it brown for 7 minutes on each side. Add salt, turmeric, garlic and ginger to the chicken. Mix to evenly combine. Add in the sliced sweet potatoes, Close the pot and cook on low heat for 20 minutes.
3. Garnish with fresh chopped cilantro right before serving. Serve hot.

Nutrition Calories: 192kcal | Carbohydrates: 7.3g | Protein: 28g | Fat: 5g | Saturated Fat: 1g | Sodium: 580mg| Fiber: 0.6g

Garlic roasted Mushrooms

Ingredients:

1. 3 tablespoon balsamic vinegar
2. 2 tablespoon coconut oil
3. 3 cloves garlic, minced
4. 1 teaspoon fresh thyme, chopped
5. Salt and ground black pepper
6. 2 lb cremini mushroom

Instructions:

1. Preheat oven to 400 degrees F. In a large bowl, add in balsamic vinegar, Oil, garlic, thyme, sea salt, and black pepper, and whisk together.
2. Add in the mushroom and toss together until coated.
3. Place the mushroom on a baking sheet in a single layer. Roast for 15 minutes, stirring halfway through, until golden and tender.

Nutrition Calories: 86kcal | Carbohydrates: 6g | Protein: 3g | Fat: 5g | Saturated Fat: 3g | Sodium: 205mg| Fiber: 2g

Pumpkin soup

1. 1 large red onion, chopped
2. 1 medium carrot, chopped
3. 1 medium butternut, chopped
4. 2 yellow squash, chopped
5. 1 Tablespoon olive oil
6. 1 teaspoon basil
7. 2 teaspoons garlic, minced
8. 1 tablespoon ground ginger, minced
9. 1/2 teaspoon salt
10. 1 teaspoon turmeric
11. 2-3 cups water or broth
12. 1 can coconut milk
13. 1/4 cup cilantro, chopped
14. 3 Tablespoons shredded coconut
15. 1 lime, quartered

Instructions:

1. Heat olive oil in a large stock pot over medium heat. Add onion and herbs and cook until onions are starting to brown, about 3 minutes.
2. Add other veggies and water. Bring to a boil and then reduce to simmer and cook for 18-20 minutes until veggies are tender.
3. Add coconut milk and simmer another few minutes. Serve topped with a squeeze of lime juice, chopped cilantro leaves and shredded coconut.
4. You can use small amount of chopped cashews or peanuts for some crunch if you are in reintroducing stage.

Nutrition Calories: 157kcal | Carbohydrates: 23g | Protein: 6.5g | Fat: 5.4g | Saturated Fat: 2g | Sodium: 373mg| Fiber: 2g

Mediterranean Tuna Salad

1. 1/2 cup cooked artichokes, drained and diced
2. 10 olives, pitted and diced
3. 2 cans tuna, flaked
4. 2 ribs of celery, diced
5. 3 tablespoon extra-virgin olive oil
6. 2 clove of garlic, minced
7. 3 tablespoons parsley, chopped
8. 1/2 tablespoon lemon juice
9. Salt to taste

Instructions:

1. Mix all the ingredients together and serve.

Nutrition Calories: 187kcal | Carbohydrates: 9.4g | Protein: 16g | Fat: 9g | Saturated Fat: 1.5g | Sodium: 402mg| Fiber: 1g

Broccoli Beef recipe

Ingredients:

1. 1 tablespoon olive oil
2. 1/2 lb beef, sliced thin
3. 3 cloves garlic, minced
4. 1 teaspoon ginger, minced
5. 1 shallot, finely chopped
6. 2 green onions, thinly sliced
7. 2 cups of broccoli florets

Instructions:

1. Heat olive oil in a skillet over medium heat. Add the beef and cook until browned, about 8 minutes. Once done remove from pan and set aside.
2. In the same pan, add garlic, ginger, shallots and green onions. Cook about a minute. Add broccoli and cover.
3. Remove cover from pan, add beef and stir to combine, cooking about 2-3 minutes. Serve immediately.

Nutrition Calories: 330kcal | Carbohydrates: 51g | Protein: 17g | Fat: 9g | Saturated Fat: 2g | Sodium: 1090mg| Fiber: 4g

Vegan Cobb Salad

Ingredients

1. 3 heads romaine lettuce
2. 1 large corn
3. 1 cup cherry tomatoes, sliced in half
4. 1/4 red onion, diced
5. 1/2 cup coconut bacon
6. 1/2 cup radishes, quartered
7. 2/3 cup any kind of vegan dressing
8. Salt & pepper, to taste
9. Fresh chopped parsley, to garnish

Instructions:

1. In individual large bowls, add the romaine and arrange the tomatoes, radishes, avocado, vegan bacon, corn and red onion over top.
2. Drizzle with dressing and sprinkle of salt and pepper.

Nutrition Calories: 307kcal | Carbohydrates: 3.6g | Protein: 23g | Fat: 22g | Saturated Fat: 8g | Sodium: 443mg| Fiber: 2.1g

Roasted Sweet Potato

1. 2 tablespoon extra-virgin olive oil
2. 2 cup Sweet potatoes, peeled and chopped to about 1" cubes
3. 1 teaspoon ground sage
4. 1/2 teaspoon sea salt

Instructions:

1. Preheat oven to 350 degrees. In a large mixing bowl, toss all ingredients until cubes are evenly coated. Put the sweet potatoes onto a parchment roasting pan. Shake the pan side-to-side to ensure that spuds are in a single, even layer.
2. Bake for 25-30 minutes, make sure they don't burn. Serve.

Nutrition Calories: 110kcal | Carbohydrates: 20.7g | Protein: 2g | Fat: 2.4g | Saturated Fat: 1g | Sodium: 36mg| Fiber: 3.3g

Vichyssoise

1. 3 leeks
2. 2 tablespoons margarine
3. 2 cups potatoes, chopped
4. 2 cups vegetable stock
5. 1½ cups Coconut Milk
6. ¾ teaspoon salt
7. Pepper, to taste
8. Chives, for garnish

Instructions:

1. Trim off the green tops of the leeks and slice lengthwise. In a saucepan over medium low heat melt the margarine. Add the leeks and cook, stirring frequently for about 10 minutes or until leeks have become tender.
2. Add potatoes and stock, bring to a boil. Reduce heat to low and cover pot, simmering for 30 minutes until potatoes are tender. Allow to cool a bit and puree in a blender.
3. Add milk, salt, and pepper and blend to mix. Allow soup to chill before serving. Top with chopped or whole chives.

Nutrition Calories: 382kcal | Carbohydrates: 53g | Protein: 12g | Fat: 14g | Saturated Fat: 8g | Sodium: 680mg| Fiber: 6.2g

Kale and chicken salad

1. 1 pound boneless, skinless chicken breasts
2. 4-5 sprigs parsley
3. 1 bay leaf
4. Pomegranate arils
5. 2 clove garlic
6. kosher salt
7. 1 teaspoon black peppercorns
8. 1 bunch kale
9. 1/4 cup extra-virgin olive oil
10. 2 tablespoons fresh lemon juice
11. 1 tablespoon balsamic vinegar
12. 1 teaspoon brown sugar

Instructions:

1. Poach the Chicken, Rinse off the chicken breasts. Fill a medium stockpot with water and add the herbs, bay leaf, 1 clove garlic, salt and peppercorns to the pot. Bring the water to a boil and add the chicken breasts.
2. Return the water to a boil and then lower heat to medium. Simmer for 5 minutes. Remove the pot from the heat, cover with a lid and keep the chicken in the hot water for another 15 to 20 minutes or until cooked through. Remove the chicken from the poaching liquid and shred, slice or cut. Set aside to cool.
3. Meanwhile, Make the Salad Step 4 Wash the kale, remove stems and chop into bite-sized pieces. In a large bowl, combine the kale with chicken. Set aside.
4. In another bowl, whisk together the olive oil, lemon juice, balsamic vinegar, remaining garlic, brown sugar and season with salt and pepper.

5. Pour the dressing over the salad ingredients and toss to coat. Chill and serve.

Nutrition Calories: 165kcal | Carbohydrates: 14g | Protein: 8g | Fat: 9.4g | Saturated Fat: 2g | Sodium: 334.5mg| Fiber: 2.2g

Chicken and dumplings

Ingredients:

1. 2 chicken breasts
2. ½ cup chicken bone broth
3. 2 cups water
4. 3 cloves garlic, minced
5. 2 bay leaves
6. 3 carrots, finely chopped
7. 3 celery stalks, finely chopped
8. Salt, to taste
9. 1 teaspoon rosemary, chopped
10. ½ large shallot, finely chopped
11. ¼ cup cassava flour
12. ¼ cup avocado oil
13. 1 cup coconut milk
14. ⅛ cup parsley, chopped
15. 1 cup cassava flour
16. 1 cup cauliflower, boiled and mashed

Instructions:

1. In a large stock pot, add broth, water, chicken, salt and bay leaves. Boil for 15-20 min or until chicken is done. Remove the chicken and bay leaves, discard bay leaves and shred chicken. Set aside.
2. Add carrots and celery to the pot and boil for about 8-10 min. In a medium-sized bowl, add cauliflower and 1 cup cassava flour. Mix until all ingredients are combined. Knead with hands into a large ball. Flatten the dough into ½" thickness with a rolling pin between 2 pieces of light floured parchment paper. Cut dumplings into rectangles with a knife. Set aside.
3. In a saucepan on medium heat, saute rosemary, garlic, and shallots in about 1 tablespoon of the avocado oil. Once the

garlic begins to brown, add remaining oil and ¼ cup cassava flour to create a roux. Continue to stir until the color begins to darken slightly.

4. Add a cup or more of the cooked broth to the saucepan and reduce to low. Stir until mixture is combined into a thick slurry. Add the prepared sauce mixture, chicken, and coconut milk to the pot of broth and vegetables. Bring to a boil once again and add dumplings one by one, gently stirring occasionally until dumplings are cooked. Top with fresh parsley and serve.

Nutrition Calories: 280kcal | Carbohydrates: 21g | Protein: 14g | Fat: 13g | Saturated Fat: 3g | Sodium: 1120mg| Fiber: 5g

Mushroom Spinach Soup

1. 1 tablespoon coconut oil
2. 2 cups cremini mushrooms, sliced
3. 6 cloves garlic, minced
4. 3 sprigs thyme
5. Salt, to taste
6. 2 tablespoon coconut vinegar
7. 1 cup bone broth
8. ¼ cup coconut cream
9. 1 cup cauliflower rice
10. 3 handful of baby spinach

Instructions:

1. Heat the oil over medium heat in a medium pot. Once it begins to brown add in the garlic, mushrooms, thyme and seasonings. Saute, stirring often, until aromatic, about 8 minutes.
2. Add in the coconut vinegar and deglaze the pan. Add in the broth and coconut cream and bring to a simmer. Stir in the cauliflower rice and spinach and cook here for 5 minutes until tender. Serve and enjoy.

Nutrition Calories: 200kcal | Carbohydrates: 21g | Protein: 7g | Fat: 11g | Saturated Fat: 3g | Sodium: 397mg| Fiber: 3.3g

Glazed Salmon

Ingredients:

1. 1 pound salmon, cut into 3 fillets
2. ½ cup coconut aminos
3. ¼ cup honey
4. 2 tablespoons apple cider vinegar
5. 1 teaspoon ginger, minced
6. 2 cloves garlic, minced
7. 1 tablespoon sesame oil
8. green onions and cilantro, to garnish

Instructions:

1. Combine number2 to 7 ingredients in a small saucepan and bring to a simmer. Cook, stirring occasionally, for about 12-15 minutes, until thick and reduced slightly. Remove from the heat and set aside to cool.
2. While sauce is cooling, prepare the salmon. Move cleaned and dried salmon let to a large bowl. Add 1/4 cup of cooled marinade and turn to coat.
3. Once coated, turn the fish to that the flesh side is down and move to the refrigerator to marinate for at least 30 minutes, or up to overnight. Set the rest of the teriyaki sauce aside.
4. When ready to cook, preheat the oven to 450. Once the salmon is ready, brush off any excess marinade and move to a baking tray lined with parchment paper lightly coated with oil.
5. Bake, flesh side up, for about 10-15 minutes, until just about. Turn the oven up to broil and brush the salmon with some of the reserved marinade. Return to the oven and broil for about 2 or 3 minutes, watching it carefully so it doesn't burn.
6. Remove from the oven and top with some cilantro and green onions. Serve alongside a nice green vegetable, and the reserved teriyaki sauce.

Nutrition Calories: 290kcal | Carbohydrates: 37g | Protein: 20g | Fat: 7g | Saturated Fat: 1g | Sodium: 460mg| Fiber: 4g

Fruit Salad with Orange dressing

1. 1 ½ cups strawberries, diced
2. 1 cup kiwi, diced
3. 1 cup mango, diced
4. ½ cup green grapes, halved
5. 1 cup blueberries
6. ½ cup purple grapes, halved
7. 1 teaspoon lime zest
8. 1 tablespoon lime juice
9. 2 tablespoon orange juice
10. 1 tablespoon honey
11. ½ tablespoon fresh mint, minced

Instructions:

1. In a large bowl, combine strawberries, mango, kiwi, green grapes, blueberries, and purple grapes. Stir to combine.
2. In a small jar or bowl, whisk together lime zest, lime juice, orange juice, honey, and mint. Stir until well combined. Pour over your fruit salad immediately, or store covered in the refrigerator until ready to drizzle over salad.

Nutrition Calories: 160kcal | Carbohydrates: 38g | Protein: 3g | Fat: 1g | Saturated Fat: 0.4g | Sodium: 34mg| Fiber: 3g

Caramelized Apple

Ingredients:

1. 2 tablespoons Coconut Oil
2. 4 Apples, sliced
3. 4 tablespoons Maple Syrup
4. ½ tablespoon Ground Cinnamon
5. Salt, to taste

Instructions:

1. Melt oil in a medium skillet over high heat. Add the apples to the pan. Saute in the pan while stirring occasionally until golden brown, about 5 minutes total. Stirring occasionally.
2. Stir in syrup, cinnamon and salt then reduce heat to medium. Simmer until apples are soft, about 5 minutes. Stirring occasionally. Serve warm.

Nutrition Calories: 211kcal | Carbohydrates: 39g | Protein: 1g | Fat: 7g | Saturated Fat: 6g | Sodium: 294mg| Fiber: 5g

Steak Fajitas

1. 1 ½ lb flank steak
2. ½ teaspoon onion powder
3. ½ teaspoon garlic powder
4. ½ teaspoon cumin
5. 1 lime, zested
6. 2 lime, juiced
7. ¼ cup avocado oil
8. 1/3 cup coconut aminos
9. Salt, to taste
10. 1 teaspoon red pepper flakes
11. ¼ cup bone broth
12. Veggies like, sliced onion, zucchini and jalapeno
13. Avocado and cilantro, to top

Instructions

1. In a small bowl, Combine Ingredients from 2-11 together using a whisk. Transfer the marinade to a gallon zip lock bag and add the flank steak. Shake or combine well to ensure that marinade is evenly incorporated. Let it marinade for at least 1 hour.
2. Heat a large cast iron pan up on medium-high heat. Remove the flank steak from the bag and place on a cutting board. Reserve the marinade and set aside.
3. Gently place the steak into the pan and let cook for 4-5 minutes. Flip over and cook for another 4-5 minutes. Remove from the pan and let rest for 10 minutes.
4. Meanwhile cook the vegetables. Pour some oil in the pan. Add vegetables and cook for 8-10 minutes until soft and cooked through. Turn off the heat.
5. Slice the steak against the grain and layer on top of cooked vegetables. Top off with sliced avocado, jalapeno, and fresh cilantro. Enjoy!

Nutrition Calories: 478kcal | Carbohydrates: 26g | Protein: 41g | Fat: 23g | Saturated Fat: 5g | Sodium: 870mg| Fiber: 7g

Oatmeal Porridge

1. 2 Yellow Squash
2. ½ Apple
3. 3 tablespoon full-fat Coconut Milk
4. 1 teaspoon Maca Powder
5. ¼ teaspoon Cinnamon
6. ½ teaspoon Vanilla Extract
7. ½ teaspoon Honey
8. Toppings: sliced apples, pomegranate arils etc.

Instructions:

1. Peel the squash, cut them in half lengthwise and remove the seeds. Cut the apple in half and remove the core.
2. Grate the squash and apple halves transfer in a medium size sauce pan. Add in the coconut milk, maca powder, cinnamon, vanilla and honey and mix well.
3. When the mixture is well combined, turn on the stove and cook on medium heat for about 10 minutes, mixing occasionally.
4. Transfer your porridge in a bowl. Garnish your porridge with all the toppings and enjoy lukewarm!

Nutrition Calories: 201kcal | Carbohydrates: 19g | Protein: 8g | Fat: 12g | Saturated Fat: 6g | Sodium: 20mg| Fiber: 5g

Chicken Noodle Soup

Ingredients:

1. 2 tablespoon Extra Virgin Olive Oil
2. 1 Medium Onion, Finely Chopped
3. 3 Cloves Garlic, minced
4. 1 Large Carrot, cut Into ½ Inch thick Slices
5. 2 Large Celery Ribs, Cut Into ½ Inch thick Slices
6. 1/4 teaspoon each of Ground Thyme, Dried Basil and Dried Oregano
7. 1/2 teaspoon Dried Dill
8. 8 Cup homemade Chicken Stock
9. 2 Large spiralized Zucchini
10. 1 ½ Cup Shredded Cooked Chicken
11. Salt and Pepper to taste
12. 2 tablespoon Parsley, Chopped

Instructions:

1. Prepare the chicken broth and shredded chicken and set aside. Chop the onions, carrot, and celery, spiralized zucchini and set aside
2. Add the olive oil to a large stock pan and heat over medium heat. Add the onions, carrots, celery, and garlic. Cook for about 6 minutes, or until celery and onions are tender, stirring frequently.
3. Add the chicken broth, shredded chicken, spiralized zucchini, thyme, basil, oregano, and dill. Bring to u boll and boil 10 to15 minutes, or until the zucchini and carrots are tender.
4. Add the parsley, then the salt and pepper to taste. Serve Hot.

Nutrition Calories: 135kcal | Carbohydrates: 8g | Protein: 12g | Fat: 7g | Saturated Fat: 1g | Sodium: 173mg| Fiber: 2g

Grilled Chicken Coleslaw

Ingredients:

1. 2 large chicken breasts
2. 1 tablespoon olive oil
3. ¼ cup white cabbage, sliced
4. ¼ cup red cabbage, sliced
5. 1/8 cup carrots, sliced
6. 2 tablespoons coconut cream
7. 1 teaspoon fresh lime juice
8. Cilantro, to garnish
9. Salt, to taste

Instructions:

1. Preheat the oven to 355°F. Pat the chicken breasts dry with paper towels and season with salt.
2. Heat the olive oil in a pan and grill the chicken on both sides until golden. Transfer the chicken onto a baking tray and cook for 10-12 minutes.
3. Meanwhile, combine the cabbage and carrots in a bowl. Dice the cooked chicken and add to the coleslaw. Garnish with parsley and serve.

Nutrition Calories: 109kcal | Carbohydrates: 2.8g | Protein: 7g | Fat: 8.4g | Saturated Fat: 2g | Sodium: 268mg| Fiber: 1g

Lamb Chops

Ingredients:

1. 2 pounds lamb loin, thick cut
2. 4 cloves garlic, minced
3. 1 tablespoon fresh rosemary, chopped
4. Salt, to taste
5. Zest of 1 lemon
6. ¼ cup olive oil

Instructions:

1. Combine the garlic, rosemary, salt, lemon zest and olive oil in a measuring cup. Pour the marinade over the lamb chops, making sure to flip them over to cover them completely. Cover and marinate the chops in the fridge for at least 1 hour, or as overnight.
2. Grill the lamb chops on medium heat for 7-10 minutes. Allow the lamb chops to rest on a plate covered with foil for 5 minutes before serving.

Nutrition Calories: 160kcal | Carbohydrates: 1g | Protein: 24g | Fat: 7g | Saturated Fat: 2.7g | Sodium: 56.1mg| Fiber: 0g

DESSERTS & SNACKS

(by Chef Amina Subramani)

Cassava Flour Pancake

Ingredients:

1. 1 cup Cassava Flour
2. 1/4 cup Tapioca Starch
3. 1 teaspoon Cream of Tartar
4. 1/2 teaspoon Baking Soda
5. 1/4 teaspoon Sea Salt
6. 1 cup + 1/8 cup Coconut Milk
7. 1/3 cup Banana, mashed
8. 1 ½ tablespoon Apple Cider Vinegar
9. 2 tablespoon Coconut Sugar
10. 1 teaspoon Vanilla Extract
11. Coconut oil

Instructions:

1. Mix all of the ingredients in a large bowl and mix until smooth, about 30 seconds.
2. Heat a skillet over medium heat. Add a small amount of coconut oil to the pan, swirl around to cover.
3. Spoon 1-2 large spoonful of batter into the pan to form a pancake, and repeat until you run out of space. Cook for 3 minutes and then flip and cook for 3 minutes more. Top with raw honey and fresh fruits if desired.

Nutrition Calories: 187kcal | Carbohydrates: 29.3g | Protein: 2g | Fat: 7g | Saturated Fat: 2g | Sodium: 223mg| Fiber: 1.3g

Pumpkin Pie

1. 1 AIP Pie crust, homemade or store bought
2. 1 (15 oz) can pumpkin purée
3. ¼ cup pure maple syrup
4. 2 tablespoon molasses
5. 2 tablespoon cassava flour
6. 1 teaspoon cinnamon
7. ½ teaspoon ground cloves
8. ¼ teaspoon ground ginger
9. 1 teaspoon vanilla
10. 1 tablespoon gelatine
11. 1 (14 oz) heavy coconut cream

Instructions:

1. Preheat oven to 350 degrees F. Make pie crust dough according to the instructions.
2. Meanwhile, Combine pumpkin, syrup, molasses, flour, cinnamon, cloves, ginger, and vanilla. Set aside.
3. Place the coconut cream in a small saucepan with no heat under the pan. Sprinkle gelatin over it. Let sit to soak in for 5 minutes.
4. Heat the pan over medium-high heat, whisking until all gelatin has dissolved, about 1 minute. Let cool for only 5 minutes, whisking occasionally.
5. Stir the coconut cream mixture into the pumpkin mixture. When it is well-combined, pour into prepared/cooled pie shell. Refrigerate until set, at least one hour.

Nutrition Calories: 342kcal | Carbohydrates: 68g | Protein: 6g | Fat: 12g | Saturated Fat: 6g | Sodium: 52mg| Fiber: 15g

Ginger Cookies

1. ¾ cup Palm Shortening
2. 1 tablespoon Molasses
3. ¼ cup Maple Sugar
4. ¾ teaspoon Vanilla Powder
5. ¾ cup Arrowroot Starch
6. ¼ cup Cassava Flour
7. 2 tablespoon Gelatin
8. 1 teaspoon Baking Soda
9. 1/2 teaspoon Cream of Tartar
10. Salt, to taste
11. 1 teaspoon Ground Cinnamon
12. 2 teaspoons Ground Ginger

Instructions:

1. Preheat the oven to 350 degrees. Rub one tablespoon of palm shortening over a large Baking sheet.
2. Combine the wet ingredients into large mixing bowl then using a hand held mixer, cream the shortening and molasses.
3. Combine all the dry ingredients into a small mixing bowl and the stir to combine then pour it into the large mixing bowl of wet ingredients. Stir to combine.
4. Make 12 balls of dough and place them on the baking sheet. Using the bottom of a glass, gently push down on each ball.

Nutrition Calories: 163kcal | Carbohydrates: 11.4g | Protein: 1g | Fat: 13g | Saturated Fat: 3g | Sodium: 192mg| Fiber: 0.5g

Banana Pudding

1. 2 large ripe bananas
2. 3 tablespoon arrowroot starch
3. 2 cups full-fat coconut milk
4. ½ teaspoon vanilla powder
5. Salt, to taste
6. 1 tablespoon coconut sugar
7. Sliced bananas

Instructions:

1. Place all ingredients in a blender and blend until smooth. Transfer to saucepan and heat on the stove over medium high heat until the mixture starts boiling.
2. Lower the heat the medium and simmer for 10 more minutes until thickened to a syrup mixture. It will thicken more as it cools.
3. Remove from heat and place in the refrigerator to cool for at 3 hours. Stir well. Serve alone, or layered with sliced bananas and vegan vanilla wafers

Nutrition Calories: 282kcal | Carbohydrates: 20g | Protein: 3g | Fat: 23g | Saturated Fat: 20g | Sodium: 131mg| Fiber: 4g

Lemon Blueberry Muffins

Ingredients:

1. ½ cup coconut milk
2. 5 tablespoon honey
3. ¼ cup lemon juice
4. 1 tablespoon lemon zest
5. 3 tablespoon coconut oil
6. 1 teaspoon vanilla extract
7. 2/3 cup coconut flour
8. ¼ cup arrowroot four
9. 1 teaspoon baking soda
10. Salt, to taste
11. ¼ cup water
12. 1 tablespoon gelatin
13. ¾ cup fresh blueberries

Instructions:

1. Preheat the oven to 350 degrees and line a muffin pan with parchment paper. In a large bowl combine the coconut milk, honey, lemon juice & zest, coconut oil, and vanilla. Whisk until smooth. In a medium sized bowl combine the flours, baking soda and salt together. Stir.
2. Slowly add the dry ingredients to the wet ingredients, whisking as you go. Whisk until thoroughly combined and no lumps.
3. Prepare the gelatin egg, pour the water in a small pan. Slowly sprinkle the gelatin over the water in a thin layer and allow to bloom for 2 minutes. Turn the heat to medium low to melt the gelatin and then whisk until frothy.
4. Pour the gelatin egg into the large bowl with the batter and quickly stir it in. Gently fold in the blueberries. Spoon the batter into the muffin cups filling them 3/4 of the way full.
5. Bake for 20-25 minutes until the tops are lightly golden brown. Remove from the oven and let cool in pan for 5 minutes. Then carefully move to a cooling rack and allow to cool.
6.

Nutrition Calories: 124kcal | Carbohydrates: 19g | Protein: 4g | Fat: 5.5g | Saturated Fat: 0.6g | Sodium: 236mg| Fiber: 3.8g

Banana Protein Balls

Ingredients:

1. ¼ cup ripe banana
2. ¼ cup coconut butter
3. ¼ cup coconut, shredded
4. ¼ cup coconut flour
5. ½ cup protein powder
6. ½ teaspoon cinnamon

Instructions:

1. Mix all ingredients in a food processor. When well-combined and the dough has formed, spoon out the dough and roll into balls.
2. Place on a parchment paper lined plate and store in the fridge until ready to eat.

Nutrition Calories: 117kcal | Carbohydrates: 10g | Protein: 19g | Fat: 0.4g | Saturated Fat: 0g | Sodium: 94.7mg| Fiber: 1g

Cinnamon Apple Bars

1. ½ cup tiger nut flour
2. ½ cup raisins
3. 1/3 cup coconut, shredded
4. Salt, to taste
5. 1 teaspoon cinnamon
6. ¼ teaspoon ground clove
7. 1 ripe plantain, Riced
8. 1 small apple, peeled, shredded (about 1/2 cup)
9. 1 tablespoon pure maple syrup
10. Coconut oil, for greasing pan

Instructions:

1. Preheat oven to 350°. In a large mixing bowl, combine tiger nut flour, raisins, salt, cinnamon, and ground clove.
2. Add Riced plantain, apple and maple syrup. Mix well. Grease a baking dish with oil.
3. Press the mixture evenly into the dish. Bake for 30 minutes. Cool and cut.

Nutrition Calories: 190kcal | Carbohydrates: 28g | Protein: 5g | Fat: 8g | Saturated Fat: 0.5g | Sodium: 40mg| Fiber: 3g

Cantaloupe Sorbet

1. 4 cups cubed cantaloupe
2. 2 tablespoon lemon juice
3. 1 tablespoon maple syrup

1. Cut the cantaloupe into cubes, Freeze for at least 2 hours.
2. Add the frozen cantaloupe cubes into the food processor and process until crumbly in texture.
3. Add lemon juice and maple syrup and pulse until incorporated. Scoop it with a spoon or an ice cream scooper. Enjoy right away or store in the freezer in an airtight container.

Nutrition Calories: 68kcal | Carbohydrates: 17g | Protein: 2g | Fat: 1g | Saturated Fat: 1g | Sodium: 35mg| Fiber: 2g

Coconut Date Balls

Ingredients:

1. 24 pitted dates
2. 3 tablespoon boiling water
3. 1/2 cup unsweetened shredded coconut

Instructions:

1. Boil water and add 3 tablespoon to shallow dish with pitted dates inside, just enough to soak up some water. Let dates soak for about 10 minutes.
2. Empty the dates into a food processor and run until dates are fully chopped and almost become paste-like.
3. Form chopped dates into small balls and roll them in a plate of shredded coconut. Place the coconut date balls in the fridge and let harden for about an hour. Enjoy!

Nutrition Calories: 87kcal | Carbohydrates: 17g | Protein: 1g | Fat: 1.8g | Saturated Fat: 1.3g | Sodium: 45mg| Fiber: 1g

Avocado Fudge

Dry Ingredients:

1. 1/3 cup green banana flour
2. 1/3 cup carob powder
3. 2 tablespoon collagen
4. Salt, to taste
5. ½ teaspoon baking soda

Wet Ingredients:

1. 2 Medium avocados
2. 1/3 cup unsweetened applesauce
3. 3 tablespoon maple syrup
4. 1 teaspoon vanilla

Instructions:

1. Mix dry ingredients in a bowl, set aside. Mix wet ingredients in a separate bowl. Add dry ingredients to wet ingredients, and mix until combined.
2. Place batter onto a parchment lined glass pan, and spread with a spatula until approximately an inch thick. Bake at 375 for 25 minutes.
3. Allow to cool completely. Store in refrigerator. Enjoy!

Nutrition Calories: 98kcal | Carbohydrates: 15g | Protein: 1g | Fat: 5g | Saturated Fat: 3g | Sodium: 73mg| Fiber: 1g

DRINKS & SMOOTHIES

(by Chef Amina Subramani)

Pumpkin Smoothie

1. ¾ cup coconut milk
2. ½ cup pumpkin puree
3. ½ of a small avocado
4. 1 teaspoon cinnamon
5. 1 tablespoon maple syrup
6. ½ teaspoon vanilla extract
7. 1 tablespoon coconut butter
8. 1 cup ice cubes, optional

Instructions:

1. Combine all ingredients in a blender and blend. Add water or ice cubes to reach desired Consistency.

Nutrition Calories: 155kcal | Carbohydrates: 29g | Protein: 5.3g | Fat: 3g | Saturated Fat: 1.7g | Sodium: 328mg| Fiber: 4g

Homemade Apple Cider

Ingredients:

1. 3 large apples, chopped
2. 6 cups water
3. 1 tablespoon cinnamon
4. 1 teaspoon cloves

Instructions:

1. Roughly chop apples. Add everything to a high powered blender and blend about 1-2 minutes, it will turn brown.
2. Strain cider through a fine mesh strainer lined with cheesecloth. Serve hot or cold.

Nutrition Calories: 110kcal | Carbohydrates: 28g | Protein: 3g | Fat: 18g | Saturated Fat: 8g | Sodium: 603mg| Fiber: 7g

Avocado Green Smoothie

Ingredients:

1. ½ ripe avocado
2. 1 ripe banana
3. ½ cup coconut milk
4. 1 handful of greens of your choice (spinach, kale, chard, broccoli)
5. 1 cup ice cubes

Instructions:

1. Place the avocado, banana, ice cubes and coconut milk into the blender.
2. Top with the greens of your choice. Blend until smooth.

Nutrition Calories: 186kcal | Carbohydrates: 12.5g | Protein: 7g | Fat: 13g | Saturated Fat: 2g | Sodium: 42.8mg| Fiber: 3g

Ginger Lemon Water

Ingredients:

1. 1 cup boiling water
2. ½ lemon, squeezed
3. ½ lemon, cut into slices
4. 3 thin slices of ginger
5. Honey to taste

Instructions:

1. Place all the ingredients into a cup. Let rest for 5 minutes and serve.

Nutrition Calories: 60kcal | Carbohydrates: 11g | Protein: 2g | Fat: 1g | Saturated Fat: 0g | Sodium: 2mg| Fiber: 1g

Coconut Blueberry Smoothie

Ingredients:

1. ½ cup Coconut Milk
2. 3 Large Kale leaves, chopped
3. 1 cup of frozen blueberries

Instructions:

1. Place all the ingredients together in a blender. Blend until smooth. Top with some blueberries and mint leaves.

Nutrition Calories: 238kcal | Carbohydrates: 27.6g | Protein: 10g | Fat: 7g | Saturated Fat: 3g | Sodium: 107.1mg| Fiber: 10g

Hot chocolate

1. 2 tablespoon carob powder
2. 2 cups coconut milk
3. 1 tablespoon coconut cream
4. ½ teaspoon maple syrup or honey

Instructions:

1. Add coconut milk to a small sauce pan and begin to heat on medium-low heat for about 4 minutes.
2. Add in coconut cream and whisk until combined and melted. Stir in carob powder, maple syrup and whisk vigorously until there are not more clumps.
3. Top with extra coconut cream if desired, and enjoy!

Nutrition Calories: 147kcal | Carbohydrates: 26g | Protein: 1g | Fat: 4g | Saturated Fat: 0.5g | Sodium: 200mg| Fiber: 1g

Green Gazpacho

1. 2 cucumbers
2. 1 medium white onion
3. 1 bell pepper, green
4. 1 clove garlic
5. 1 medium avocado
6. 1/4 cup fresh parsley
7. 1/4 cup fresh cilantro
8. 2 tablespoon olive oil
9. Salt, to taste
10. 1 tablespoon lemon juice
11. water

Instructions:

1. Slice the cucumber in half lengthwise. Scrape the seeds out with a spoon and then chop the cucumber into chunks. Remove the seeds from the bell pepper and also cut it into chunks. Dice the onion.
2. Add the cucumber, bell pepper, onion, and garlic to a food processor. Process until fully combined and minced
3. Add the fresh leaves to the food processor along with olive oil and the flesh from the avocado. Puree until smooth.
4. Add some water, one tablespoon of lemon juice, and one teaspoon of salt. Puree until smooth again. Serve immediately or chill until ready to eat.

Nutrition Calories: 214kcal | Carbohydrates: 13.5g | Protein: 3g | Fat: 18g | Saturated Fat: 8g | Sodium: 603mg| Fiber: 7g

Cranberry Juice

Ingredients:

1. 8 cups Cranberries, fresh or frozen
2. 1 cup Honey
3. 8 cups Water

Instructions:

1. Add cranberries and water to a large saucepan. Bring to a boil, stirring occasionally. Reduce heat to low and simmer for 15-20 minutes, stirring occasionally.
2. Place a fine mesh strainer over a bowl and pour the berries into it. Discard the berries. Pour the honey into the bowl with the hot juice. Stir until the honey is dissolved completely.
3. Allow the juice to cool. Serve and enjoy.

Nutrition Calories: 177kcal | Carbohydrates: 47g | Protein: 1g | Fat: 1g | Saturated Fat: 0g | Sodium: 13mg| Fiber: 4g

Green Detox Drink

Ingredients:

1. 5 oz (140g) of kale, roughly chopped
2. 1 small green apple, core removed and roughly chopped
3. 3.5 oz celery stalks, roughly chopped
4. 1 lemon, rind and pips removed and diced
5. Generous handful mint leaves
6. 1 thumb-size piece ginger, peeled and roughly diced

Instructions:

1. Place all the ingredients into a juicer and switch the juicer on. Once done, discard the Pulp. Stir the juice well and enjoy with ice, if needed.

Nutrition Calories: 184kcal | Carbohydrates: 44g | Protein: 4.3g | Fat: 2g | Saturated Fat: 0.5g | Sodium: 35mg| Fiber: 4.5g

Banana Coconut Smoothie

Ingredients:

1. ¾ cup coconut milk
2. 1 small frozen banana
3. 1 teaspoon honey
4. Ice cubes and Water, as needed

Instructions:

1. Combine all ingredients in a blender, and blend until smooth. Taste for sweetness then serve immediately.

Nutrition Calories: 157kcal | Carbohydrates: 26g | Protein: 9g | Fat: 3g | Saturated Fat: 1.7g | Sodium: 108mg| Fiber: 1.4g

28 days Meal plan

(by Chef Amina Subramani)

Day 1

Breakfast: Pumpkin Smoothie

Lunch: Honey Garlic Chicken

Dinner: Teriyaki meatballs

Day 2:

Breakfast: Shepherd's pie

Lunch: Burrito Bowl

Dinner: Lamb Chops

Day 3:

Breakfast: Broccoli Burger

Lunch: Beef Bourguignon

Dinner: Pumpkin Pie

Day 4:

Breakfast: Mexican ground beef skillet

Lunch: chicken noodle soup

Dinner: vichyssoise

Day 5:

Breakfast: Sweet potato avocado toast

Lunch: teriyaki meatballs

Dinner: steak fajitas

Day 6:

Breakfast: Shrimp scampi with zucchini noodles

Lunch: chicken and vegetable curry

Dinner: Cassava flour naan flatbread

Day 7:

Breakfast: Lettuce burger

Lunch: chicken and dumplings

Dinner: Hot chocolate

Day 8:

Breakfast: Baked salmon

Lunch: Broccoli Beef

Dinner: Chicken noodle soup

Day 9:

Breakfast: Grilled fish tacos

Lunch: Crockpot chicken stew

Dinner: Roasted cauliflower soup

Day 10:

Breakfast: Avocado green smoothie

Lunch: Stuffed mushroom

Dinner: Grilled chicken coleslaw

Day 11:

Breakfast: Harvest Bowl

Lunch: Tuna salad

Dinner: Banana pudding

Day 12:

Breakfast: Banana coconut smoothie

Lunch: Squash pasta salad

Dinner: Lamb chops

Day 13:

Breakfast: Ginger lemon water

Lunch: Beef lettuce wrap

Dinner: Glazed salmon

Day 14:

Breakfast: Shrimp and asparagus

Lunch: Mushroom spinach soup

Dinner: Cassava flour Naan flatbread

Day 15:

Breakfast: Chicken Burrito

Lunch: Fruit salad with orange dressing

Dinner: Honey garlic Chicken

Day 16:

Breakfast: Vegetarian Chow mein

Lunch: Glazed salmon

Dinner: Shepherd's pie

Day 17:

Breakfast: Chicken Quesadilla

Lunch: Beef stir fry

Dinner: Zucchini Lasagna

Day 18:

Breakfast: Pumpkin Soup

Lunch: Chicken and dumplings

Dinner: vegan Cobb salad

Day 19:

Breakfast: Broccoli chicken casserole

Lunch: Garlic roasted mushroom

Dinner: Mushroom spinach soup

Day 20:

Breakfast: Green detox drink

Lunch: Turmeric chicken

Dinner: Cinnamon apple bars

Day 21:

Breakfast: Coconut blueberry smoothie

Lunch: cauliflower risotto

Dinner: Roasted Sweet potato

Day 22:

Breakfast: Caramelized apples

Lunch: Grilled fish tacos

Dinner: Cranberry Juice

Day 23:

Breakfast: Chicken Alfredo

Lunch: Cauliflower fried rice

Dinner: Steak Fajitas

Day 24:

Breakfast: Green gazpacho

Lunch: chicken and vegetable curry

Dinner: kale and chicken salad

Day 25:

Breakfast: Pumpkin smoothie

Lunch: Shrimp scampi with zucchini noodles

Dinner: Cassava flour naan flatbread

Day 26:

Breakfast: Burrito Bowl

Lunch: Spinach chicken soup

Dinner: coconut date balls

Day 27:

Breakfast: AIP oatmeal porridge

Lunch: Shrimp and asparagus

Dinner: Mexican ground beef skillet

Day 28:

Breakfast: Cassava flour pancake

Lunch: Chicken and dumplings

Dinner: Teriyaki meatballs

Conclusion:

(by Researcher Tracy Cooper)

Choosing to adopt this protocol means consciously choosing a detoxification path thanks to a choice: CLEAN FOOD.
This road may initially seem uphill, it may seem not worth it … after all, any one of us thinks that food is one of the pleasures of life!!
You will have to remain lucid and focused on the final goal, because, especially the initial phase, will be a phase of renunciation, sacrifice, and great mental test; it will be your determination, your desire to "lighten" your body from everything toxic for you, to bring you the physical and mental benefits. Therefore, the approach you will adopt will help you to believe in this project and to achieve the desired results.
Unfortunately, there are more than 80 different autoimmune diseases,
Below is a shortlist of diseases associated with impaired intestinal permeability (leaky gut) with an autoimmune response:

- Rheumatoid arthritis
- Celiac disease
- Type 1 diabetes
- Hypothyroidism
- Crohn's disease
- Narcolepsy
- Psoriasis
- Multiple sclerosis
- Hashimoto's thyroiditis
- Vitiligo….

All of these diseases share a common cause: damage to the intestinal mucosa that makes the intestines permeable and causes the response of an autoimmune disease.
A healthy intestine allows the absorption of nutrients and creates a barrier against toxins and allergenic substances by blocking their passage. When the intestine becomes permeable, the mucous membrane of the intestinal defensive barrier tears, enlarging the meshes, and the toxins overcome the intestinal barrier and pour into the blood causing various types of disorders. Intestinal permeability

is caused by various factors, often due to a harmful diet: among the main culprits are cereals which, as we know, contain lectins, legumes and nightshades also contain saponins, substances that can cause intestinal permeability.

For those who are already following the Paleo diet and suffer from an autoimmune disease or for those interested in deep detoxification of the body, there is a further exclusion of foods allowed by the Paleo diet.

Research is constantly evolving, there are no guarantees that the food restrictions will cure autoimmune diseases, there are testimonies that make us think so and we can certainly deduce that by feeding ourselves with "real food", with poorly processed foods, we can guarantee our body a more complete and rich supply of nutrients, essential to produce the necessary energy and maintain a good level of psycho-physical health.

For all these reasons, the elimination diet must be followed for at least 3-6 weeks, only then proceed with the slow and gradual reintroduction of one food at a time to find one's balance and achieve as much as possible a varied, complete, and nutritious diet.

What should be eliminated?

In detail, a specific list of items to avoid:

- Gluten (wheat, rye, barley, spelled, Kamut, spelled, triticale, couscous, bulgur, bran, seitan).
- Dairy product.
- Lectins contained in legumes and cereals.
- Saponins are contained in legumes and cereals, including pseudocereals such as quinoa and amaranth.
- Solanaceae *: tomatoes, potatoes, peppers, aubergines, goji berries, pepper.
- Phytic acid: dried fruit and oil seeds * (to be evaluated case by case).
- Spices derived from seeds and fruits (turmeric, cinnamon, and ginger could be tolerated).
- Eggs *, in particular the egg white.
- Alcohol in general.
- Caffeine, theine, theobromine (coffee and drinks that contain it, tea, chocolate, and cocoa).
- Sugar, artificial sweeteners.

- Hydrogenated / trans vegetable fats, refined vegetable oils.
- Preservatives, dyes, thickeners.

So, during this phase of elimination, what can I feed on?

- Dark green leafy vegetables, vegetables from the cruciferous family (cauliflower, broccoli, cabbage).
- Vegetables rich in sulfur such as garlic, onions, asparagus.
- Colored vegetables, roots (carrots, turnips, celeriac).
- Batata or American potato, cassava, pumpkin.
- Fresh fruit (especially berries, lime, lemon), without exaggerating!
- Banana, plane tree.
- Avocado and coconut (good sources of monounsaturated fats).
- Fish (caught in the Mediterranean or the cold seas - avoiding those of African and Asian origin).
- Grass-fed animal meat or free-range poultry (or organic).
- Offal of grass-fed animals.
- Bone broth.
- PDO raw ham.
- Collagen proteins
- Extra virgin olive oil.
- Unpasteurized apple vinegar.
- Whole wheat or Himalayan pink salt.
- Rosemary, thyme, sage, basil, aromatic herbs.
- Extra virgin coconut oil, unrefined.
- Coconut butter.
- Coconut flour (absorbs liquids a lot).
- Carob flour (not carob seeds).
- Arrowroot (works as a thickener and binder).
- Cassava or tapioca flour (derives from a tuber for which a good source of carbohydrates).
- Chufa flour (naturally sweet, somewhat reminiscent of almonds and hazelnuts).
- Local honey, coconut sugar (from coconut blossom), dates as sweeteners in controlled doses.

So, why not try the Anti-Inflammatory diet?

Eat clean!!

When deciding to adopt the Autoimmune Protocol, food choices will focus on consuming nutrients and taking dietary supplements to promote healing and provide the body with the tools and resources it needs to stop sticking and help repair damaged tissue. and then return to health.

As mentioned, a few lines above, it will not be a walk in the park, it will be challenging, and it will take perseverance and commitment. But following our advice to the letter, we cannot tell you that you will recover at all, but you will experience real benefits for your body, which will allow you to detoxify your body, and recover the joy of eating.

Our suggestions could be a way to continue to cultivate your passion for cooking (so it was for us, in creating them !!), and at the same time get closer to this protocol that is still not too well known, but which scientific studies are demonstrating its effectiveness in restoring "normality" and dignity to your life.

Keep your hunger alive in the kitchen and outside the kitchen!!

Eat clean!!

Enjoy the diet, enjoy new life!!

Amina Subramani & Tracy Cooper

Thank you for reading this book. If you enjoyed it, please visit the site where you purchased it and write a brief review. your feedback is important to me and will help other readers decide whether to read the book too. Thank you

AIP DIET

COOKBOOK

SECTION 1: A GENERAL INTRODUCTION TO AUTO-IMMUNE PROTOCOL

WHAT IS AIP (AUTO-IMMUNE PROTOCOL)

Dear reader, thank you for taking your time to read this book. Before we get to cooking, I believe that it is best to understand the reasons why we want to embark on the journey of cooking AIP diets and to have in-depth knowledge about the meaning of AIP itself.

Unlike many other books that focus solely on the food and nutritional aspect, I want to use this book as a resource of research for knowing more about Autoimmune diseases and disorders.

AIP is a systematic approach to chronic disease treatment, the Autoimmune Protocol focuses on supplying the body with the nutritional elements needed for immune control, gut health, hormone regulation, and tissue healing while eliminating toxic stimuli from both diet and lifestyle. The AIP diet aims to help avoid processed and refined foods and empty calories, substituting it with healthy and full nutrition. As these are major immune modulators, the AIP lifestyle promotes adequate sleep, stress control, and exercise.

It is possible to see foods as having two different constituents within them: those that foster wellbeing (nutrients) and those that threaten health (like toxic compounds). Certain foods are generally necessary for a healthy diet because they contain lots of nutrients that aid good health and zero to little harmful nutrients or constituents. Some examples of these beneficial foods are organic meats and livers, fish, and most legumes and vegetables. Other foods are apparent failures since they have a relative lack of components that promote wellbeing and are riddled with toxic compounds, with gluten-containing wheat, peanuts, and some soy products being good examples. But in between these two extremes, several foods fall into the undifferentiated sections. For instance, tomatoes have some beneficial constituents, but they also sometimes contain some compounds that are so effective in energizing the immune system, so much that they have been investigated for use as immune enhancers in vaccines. The key distinction between the Autoimmune Protocol and other dietary models that follow a nutrient-first approach is to draw the line between "acceptable" foods and "unacceptable" foods to get more health-promoting compounds and less inflammatory compounds in our diet when recognizing inflammation triggers. Healthier people will be able to consume foods that are less-optimal than less healthy people. Like a better version of other evidence-based dietary templates, you might think of the Autoimmune Protocol; it embraces only certain items that are strong winners.

To recap, The Autoimmune Protocol puts more emphasis on the most nutritionally rich foods, including organ meat (Liver etc.), fish, and vegetables, in our food supply. And the Autoimmune Protocol excludes foods that are supported by other safe diets, (like tomatoes and peppers), nuts, eggs, seeds, and alcohol, that have compounds that may trigger the immune system or damage the gut system. The Autoimmune Protocol's purpose is to supply the body with nutrients while eliminating any food that may lead to disease-triggering hormones at the same time or nutrients that disturb healing.

The AIP diet is an elimination method, as cuts out the foods that are most likely to hinder our wellbeing. Many of the foods excluded in the AIP diet can be reintroduced after a while, especially those that have nutritional significance while still having some (but not too many) potentially harmful compounds. Given your particular health issues, the AIP diet is not a prison sentence, but rather a set of guidelines filled with methods and knowledge of how your body responds to your feeding, habits, lifestyle, and your environment as well as being a good technique for healing.

A diet aimed at minimizing inflammation, discomfort, and other symptoms induced by autoimmune diseases such as celiac disease, inflammatory bowel disease (IBD), lupus, and rheumatoid arthritis is known as the Autoimmune Protocol diet (AIP diet).

In addition to the lower perception of common symptoms of autoimmune disorders, such as intestinal fatigue and swelling or joint pain, many people have chosen the AIP diet to confirm changes in the way they feel.

Yet, while research is promising on this diet, it's also limited.

The goal of the autoimmune protocol (AIP) diet is to decrease inflammation and alleviate other autoimmune disorder symptoms since some nutrients overtly trigger the immune system without plausible cause.

The AIP is also a systematic approach to wellness, including a nutritional system and a focus on lifestyle variables considered to be significant immune function, gut health, and hormone health modulators. This requires a heavy emphasis on having enough sleep, stress control, and living an active lifestyle while preventing system overload. To aim for a healthy gut, these aspects of the lifestyle we lead are most important because they have a direct impact on intestinal bacteria (getting enough sleep, trying to avoid high levels of stress, and practicing regular physical activity are all necessary components. to foster the development of a healthy and diverse intestinal microbial environment and not least to aid in the development of key probiotic strains).

Intestinal permeability is also worsened by chronic stress and overload. All essential hormone modulators are sleep, stress, and activity; insulin sensitivity, for example, is more affected by these lifestyle factors than by diet. And, most significantly, there is a clear correlation between immune function and lifestyle. Inflammation is caused by being less inadequate, feeling anxious, passive, and over-straining.

Many of the aspects that regulate the immune system are involved during sleep, and there is a close correlation between stress and sleep quality.

Furthermore, there is emerging evidence that a good sense of relationship and society as well as spending quality time in natural settings often leads to a healthy immune system.

The AIP is now backed by clinical study and evidence, building on observations gathered from over 1,000 research studies.

An increasing number of physicians, in particular specialists in functional and integrative medicine, are prescribing the AIP to their patients, contributing to the wide body of anecdotal evidence that supports the Autoimmune Protocol's effectiveness. Ongoing clinical studies to measure progress in particular autoimmune disorders with short-term AIP intervention, including research on Hashimoto's thyroiditis, is in the works. As the discoveries of more clinical trials are published, more attention is paid to diet and lifestyle, not as a supplementary approach to the management of autoimmune disorders, but as a first-line treatment path.

An autoimmune disease causes the immune system, by accident, to attack and harm healthy tissues or organs.

Psoriasis, rheumatoid arthritis, and lupus are typical examples of this type of disease.

Inflammation may be triggered by an autoimmune disorder, frequent fatigue is another common symptom of the disorder. Additional signs can include discomfort, swelling, skin lesions, and a fever, depending on the condition.

Inflammation and other symptoms of autoimmune disorders can be decreased by the AIP diet.

There are over a hundred autoimmune diseases reported and several more diseases suspected of having autoimmune causes. These two autoimmune diseases have essentially the same cause: our immune system instead of protecting us from microbes that threaten our organism assaults us and attacks our proteins, cells, and tissues.

Autoimmune disorder and its signs are dictated by what proteins, cells, and tissues are targeted. For example, Hashimoto's thyroiditis affects the thyroid gland. The tissues in your joints are attacked in the event of rheumatoid arthritis. The proteins found inside the cells that make up your skin are attacked and this process causes psoriasis.

In the present society, an autoimmune disorder is an epidemic that affects an estimated 50 million Americans. While about one-third of the risk of having an autoimmune disorder is due to genetic predisposition, the other two-thirds are from your environment, your diet, and your lifestyle. Indeed, it is widely recognized by experts that nutritional factors are the main contributors to autoimmune diseases, putting these autoimmune disorders in the same class of dietary and lifestyle-related diseases such as type 2 diabetes, cardiovascular disease, and obesity. This suggests that our food options and our life-style are the main causes of autoimmune disease. It also means that by improving how you eat and making more educated decisions about sleep, exercise, and stress, we can simply control and reverse autoimmune disease.

Why does the immune system become so disoriented that the body begins to attach itself?

The answer is Autoimmunity, as the immune system's tendency to destroy native tissues, turns out to be a relatively frequent accident. In fact, at any given time, about 30 percent of people would have detectable amounts of autoantibodies in their blood (antibodies that bind to a certain protein in our bodies instead of, or in addition to, another protein called an antigen).

This mechanism is so widespread that there are many "alarms" in our immune system to detect and suppress autoimmunity.

What happens in autoimmune disease is not only the autoimmunity accident but also the ability of the immune system to malfunction, stimuli target the immune-system and the body works against itself.

In recent decades, the number of cases of autoimmune diseases is, unfortunately, growing exponentially; the reasons are statistically a frequent interaction between your genetic predisposition and the environment in which you live, a mix of conditions that make it difficult for our immune system to understand what is useful to avoid and what, on the other hand, is necessary for our body.

AIP technique uses diet and lifestyle to manage the immune system, put an end to these attacks and give the body the chance to recover.

WHAT IS AIP DISORDER

In order to generate antibodies that kill foreign or harmful cells in our body, a well healthy immune system was built.

In individuals with autoimmune disorders, however, the immune system appears to develop antibodies that target healthy cells and tissues rather than battle dangerous cells and infections.

This can lead to several symptoms, including pain in the joints, exhaustion, stomach pain, diarrhea, brain fog, and damage to tissues and nerves.

Rheumatoid arthritis, lupus, IBD, type 1 diabetes, and psoriasis are only a few examples of autoimmune disorders.

A variety of causes, including hereditary propensity, infection, stress, inflammation, and drug use, are thought to be caused by autoimmune diseases.

Some research also indicates increased intestinal permeability may be caused by damage to the intestinal barrier. In individuals whose genetic predisposition is favorable, this "permeability" can lead to the development of some autoimmune diseases.

It is suspected that certain foods can increase the permeability of the gut, thereby raising the likelihood of leaky intestines.

The prerogative of the AIP diet is to focus on replacing these foods with nutrient-rich foods that promote good functioning of the entire digestive system and lead the intestine towards healing. The newfound intestinal health relieves inflammation and consequently all those symptoms of autoimmune diseases.

It also eliminates certain ingredients, such as gluten, which when surplus in diets can cause irregular immune responses.

Although experts agree that a leaky gut could be a possible explanation for the inflammation encountered by individuals with autoimmune disorders, they caution that a cause-and-effect connection between the two cannot be verified by current research.

Therefore, before firm assumptions can be made, further study is needed.

The idea behind the AIP diet is that it would minimize inflammation by eliminating gut-irritating foods and consuming nutrient-rich ones.

The leaky gut theory is called one hypothesis on how autoimmune conditions begin. It notes that if there is a problem with the bacterial composition of the gut of an individual, inflammatory environmental factors, such as toxins and viruses, will penetrate the intestinal wall and enter other areas of the body.

This theory's proponents claim that consuming the right foods will help prevent inflammatory symptoms, but many experts are skeptical.

Many advocates of the theory of the leaky gut claim that the AIP diet can help avoid tissue attacks by the immune system and decrease the symptoms of autoimmune diseases.

HOW DOES THE AUTOIMMUNE PROTOCOL WORK?

Continuous scientific studies, and increasingly avant-garde research suggest that there are currently 4 factors that particularly affect the immune system and in which the Autoimmune Protocol seems to have greater efficacy:

- **Density of nutrients.**

A good number of vitamins, minerals, antioxidants, essential fatty acids, and amino acids are necessary and regulate and balance the normal functioning of the immune system.

Deficiencies and imbalances in micronutrients are important players in autoimmune disease growth and progression. To correct any imbalances or deficiencies it, therefore, becomes necessary to focus on the consumption of more nutritious foods; this synergy of micronutrients will contribute to the control of the immune system, it will facilitate the development of neurotransmitters, the detoxification systems, and therefore the hormonal development.

The building blocks the body requires to repair damaged tissues are provided by a nutrient-dense diet.

- **Gut Health.**

In the development of autoimmune disorders, gut dysbiosis and leaky intestines are major players. The foods recommended under the Autoimmune Protocol encourage healthy levels of growth and a healthy range of microorganisms in the gut. Foods that irritate or damage the gut lining are discouraged while foods that help restore the function of the intestinal barrier and facilitate healing are encouraged. The Autoimmune Protocol also discusses lifestyle factors that greatly affect the health of the intestinal barrier and the microbial composition of the gut. The restoration of a healthy gut barrier and microbiome are important precursors to healing some chronic diseases because of the direct connection between gut health and immune function.

- **Regulation of hormones.**

Many hormones that interfere with the immune system are affected by what we eat, how we drink, and how much we eat. The immune system is more affected by dietary factors (such as consuming too many sugar-containing foods or eating under stress rather than intermittently eating full meals). These factors affect the malfunction of these hormones.

The diet of the Autoimmune Protocol is intended to facilitate the regulation of these hormones, thereby controlling the immune system. The amount of sleep we get, how much time we spend outdoors, how much of and what kinds of exercise we get, and how well we minimize and handle stress all have a significant effect on our bodies and the important hormones that influence the immune system.

- **Regulation of the immune system.**

Immune system control is accomplished by restoring a healthy variety and healthy amounts of gut microbes, restoring the gut's barrier function, supplying the immune system with adequate quantities of the micronutrients needed to function normally, and controlling the main hormones that then regulate the immune system in return. With the AIP diet, r Both the tools and the potential for immune regulation are created by the Autoimmune Protocol diet and lifestyle. Reductions in symptoms are compensated for by immune regulation combined with tissue healing.

In all chronic diseases, inflammation is a factor, and this is one place where the foods we consume can make a big difference. In some cases, the disease is triggered directly by an immune system that does not control itself properly; in others, inflammation is merely an aspect of the disease or a contributor to how the disease happens, but it is still a contributing factor and a concern.
Therefore it is important to understand that for those who suffer from chronic ailments, it is only by reducing inflammation that you give the immune system respite; the goal then becomes to provide the system itself with all the tools it needs, as this will help restore healthy health and the body will be "educated" again in self-management.

Equally important will be to understand that everything we eat, the quality of sleep, our general level of stress and fatigue (both mental and physical), have a great influence on the onset of inflammation. And this is a bit of the reason why chronic disorders have a statistically difficult life in the presence of a correct diet and a correct lifestyle.

Here are some common Auto-immune diseases

- Angioedema
- Rheumatoid Arthritis
- Type 1 Diabetes
- Narcolepsy
- Crohn's Disease
- Psoriasis
- Alopecia Areata
- Multiple Sclerosis
- Celiac Disease
- Lupus
- Ulcerative Colitis
- Graves' disease
- Guillain-Barre Syndrome
- Hidradenitis Suppurativa
- Autoimmune Hepatitis
- Hashimoto's Thyroiditis

For any chronic disease, food has therapeutic value, but that's not the same thing as calling food a cure. Dietary modifications can take you as far as a complete reversal of your illness, or they can delay the development of any illness.

All these are achievements that are worth celebrating. The miracle cure you're looking for may not be good food, but if it helps, it's good enough.

When choosing the autoimmune protocol, your dietary decisions are based on the consumption of food to facilitate recovery.

ADDITIONAL FACTORS THAT AID RECOVERY WITH AIP DIET

Sleep: Make sure you are sleeping well—this is essential for healing and allowing your body to restore itself. Aim for at least 8 hours of uninterrupted sleep per night—more if you can manage it.

· Stress management: Engage in at least one activity aimed at reducing your stress level every day, whether it be meditation, walking, taking a bath or anything else that helps you to relax.

· Movement: Make an effort to do one movement-based activity every day. This could be gentle exercise like yoga, qigong or walking, or more intense activity like bike riding, running or hiking.

· Sunlight exposure: It is very important to get sunlight exposure on some part of your body (it could just be your face and arms) for 20 minutes every day. This stimulates your body's production of vitamin D, which is extremely important to the healing process.

In addition to these lifestyle factors, finding a practitioner trained in functional medicine can be an invaluable part of monitoring your progress with testing as well as making individual supplement recommendations. Be sure to visit the resources section to find practitioners who integrate dietary approaches into their practices.

SECTION 2: HOW TO EAT IN THE AUTO-IMMUNE PROTOCOL

Following the AIP diet means increasing your nutrient-dense, health-promoting food intake while eliminating foods that may cause illness.

The rules on what to eat, in short, are:

Meat and offal (at least 5 times a week).

Fish and shellfish (at least 3 times a week).

Vegetables of all kinds are targeted at 8+ servings daily, with as much variety as possible.

Green vegetables with leaves (lettuce, collards, kale, spinach, celery leaves, etc.)

Colorful fruits and vegetables.

Roots, Tubers and Quash in winter (cassava, acorn squash, sweet potato, parsnip, fennel, carrots, beets, rutabaga, spaghetti squash, turnip, etc.)

Vegetables Cruciferous (Brussels sprouts, mustard greens, arugula, turnips, kale, broccoli, watercress, broccoli, cabbage)

Onions (aka alliums, onions, garlic, leek, ramps, etc.)

Vegetables from the Sea (except algae like spirulina and chlorella which are immune stimulators)

Mushrooms (and other edible fungi)

Spices and herbs

Quality meat (grass-fed, grass-raised, as wild as possible) (poultry in moderation due to high omega-6 content unless you are eating a ton of fish)

Good fats (fatty fish, avocado oil, palm oil, coconut oil, pastured/grass-fed animal fats)

Fermented/probiotic foods (fermented vegetables or fruit, water kefir, kombucha, coconut milk yogurt, coconut milk kefir, supplements).

Glycine-rich foods

Intestinal Microbiota Superfoods (bone broth, apple family, berries, high-fiber, and phytonutrient fruits and vegetables, fish, extra virgin olive oil, honey and bee products, cruciferous vegetables, tubers, mushrooms, roots, tubers, citrus, shellfish, leafy greens, alliums, fermented foods, tea).

Delete the following from your diet:

Grains

Legumes

Dairy or milk.

These sugars and fats get refined and processed.

Nuts

The Nightshade family of plants (potatoes [sweet potatoes are fine, goji berries, eggplants, ect ... all kinds of hot peppers, and spices derived from peppers, including paprika)

Eggs

Seeds

Consider these possible gluten cross-reactive foods.

Alcohol

NSAIDS (like aspirin or ibuprofen)

Sugar-free or non-nutritive sweeteners. (even stevia and monk fruit)

Food additives including emulsifiers, thickeners, and flavoring agents.

Stick to a modest amount of the following:

Fructose is fruit sugar.

Salt (using only Himalayan pink salt or Celtic gray salt --- unrefined salt)

High-glycemic-load fruits and vegetables– (remember, the AIP is not a low-carb diet).

A fatty acid-rich diet consists of omega-6 fatty acids.

Black tea and green tea.

Sugars found in nature (honey and blackstrap molasses).

Saturated fat is really healthy.

This diet is ideal for all those individuals diagnosed and certified with autoimmune diseases or suspected autoimmune diseases. When you get started, do not forget to ditch any of the traditional unhealthy foods such as wheat and dairy. Kefir is a versatile food that will help your stomach function more healthily. If you have a serious autoimmune disorder that causes additional sensitivity to food, your food choices should be carefully drafted and taken into account according to the following.

FACTORS THAT CONTRIBUTE TO A BALANCED LIFESTYLE.

As we have already repeated in the previous pages, some factors cannot be overlooked: the quality of sleep (at least 8 hours), trying to avoid or at least recognize moments of stress, to counteract it in some way (there are much mental training, meditation, yoga, tantra - which seem to bring significant benefits and relieve stress conditions), stay in contact with nature, try to have fun while respecting the circadian cycles (the day awake and in the light, the night in the dark and sleep !!), play sports, without straining the body too much, have a social life and free time to devote to hobbies (this also helps to remove tension)

Elimination and Reintroduction (E&R).

The AIP is used to restructure the diet of a person that has hormonal or imbalances due to suboptimal foods.

This diet is based on a concept of "elimination" at its heart, which works with the idea that the body ejects the cause of an illness from the system.

Many people who adopt the Autoimmune Protocol (AIP) develop an aversion to eggs, which may result in a paradoxical feeling of better health. And getting the eliminated food reintroduced again is a crucial part of your development in health. Plus, having food versatility will make your life easier by making it possible to eat in different places. You'll also be more prepared for work because you can make certain decisions quicker.

Your reintroductions will motivate you to commit to new behaviors. If you can successfully eliminate and reintroduce foods to your diet, you will be able to add new foods to your diet, getting you closer to a more diverse diet.

Please note that the current AIP is a protocol packed with scientifically tested tips for healing.

You need a mastery of the subject you're exploring and you know just how to apply it to the reading. There are a few common threads here, including adhering to your low-strain diet, having plenty of rest, and staying hydrated before you start feeling better again.

Here is a step-by-step guide to the reintroduction of foods that have been avoided during the AIP diet process of elimination.

Stage 1. Pick one food that needs to be reintroduced. Plan on the testing day to eat this food a few times a day, then stop it for 5-6 days altogether.

Stage 2. Eat a small dose of the food, such as 1 teaspoon, then wait 15 minutes for any possible reaction.

Stage 3. Finish the test and stop this food if you have any symptoms. Eat a little larger dose, such as 1 1/2 teaspoons, of the same food, wait for any possible reactions and track how you feel for the next 2 hours.

Stage 4. Terminate the test and avoid foods that cause any strong or weird reactions during this time. Eat a normal portion of the same food if no reactions arise, avoid it for 5-6 days.

Stage 5. Try to reincorporate the checked food into your diet if you have no symptoms for 5-6 days, then try to repeat this 5-stage and try to re-introduct every food that you wish to re-enter.

In all those occasions when it seems to us that the inflammation increases instead of decreasing, it is therefore recommended to avoid reintroducing food.

The results of reintroducing might not be easily noticed after a bad night's sleep during an illness or while feeling unusually depressed, or after a strenuous workout.

In addition, reintroducing foods in a specific order is often recommended.

For example, when deciding to reintroduce diary products, it would be helpful to start with diary products with the lowest concentration of lactose, such as ghee or fermented milk products.

A COMPREHENSIVE LIST OF FOOD FOR EACH REINTRODUCTION STAGE

STAGE 1:

Legumes with edible pods

Seed-based spices

Ghee from grass-fed dairy

Egg yolks

Seed-based spices

Seed and nut oils

Fruit and berry-based spices

STAGE 2:

Egg whites

Nuts (except cashews and pistachios)

Egg whites

Seeds

Butter from grass-fed dairy

Cocoa or chocolate

Alcohol (in small quantities)

STAGE 3:

Fermented raw dairy (yoghurt and kefir) from grass-fed dairy

Eggplants (aubergines)

Raw cream from grass-fed dairy

Capsicums

Paprika

Capsicums

Cashews and pistachios

Coffee

Raw cream from grass-fed dairy

STAGE 4:

Dairy products

White rice

Traditionally prepared legumes (soaked and fermented)

Potatoes

Chili peppers

Other nightshades and nightshade spices

Traditionally prepared gluten-free grains (soaked and fermented)

Tomatoes

Alcohol (in larger quantities)

Foods you have a past of severe reaction to.

Foods you are allergic to.

Once you begin reintroducing foods and learning how to gauge your reactions to them, you will start to put together a safe diet that best manages your condition. While a negative reaction to a food can be discouraging, don't discount that you may be able to tolerate that food a few months down the line as your body continues to heal. My advice is to be cautious, take it slow and, when in doubt, leave it out. Over time, you will learn to better listen to your body's language as it tells you how to discern which foods are promoting health and which ones are slowing your progress.

FOODS TO AVOID:

A framework for the basic Autoimmune Diet is the criteria for what foods should be consumed or avoided in this section, but you can and completely should include those that do not harm you or remove foods that do.

Your Autoimmune Paleo Diet will be unique to you, so modify it as you see fit.

The list of foods for AIP is very diverse. We cannot possibly list every food available, so pay attention to the families the foods fall under and add or avoid other foods in those families, as well.

Foods, Drinks, and Medications to Avoid

Most diets have rules that look really impressive with do-not-eat lists, but often it seems as if the evidence behind the instructions is lacking.

Having the knowledge of why you should eat or avoid eating certain foods often makes it easier to deny the urge of eating them.

This data is especially relevant when you follow a programme, such as the Autoimmune Diet, intended to restore the body. To understand your own autoimmune disease and why you could experience flare-ups from foods like egg yolks when someone else is not affected and the mechanisms of what happens when you eat grains or have a glass of wine are important.

Alcohol

In general, alcohol can increase intestinal permeability and increase the permeability of the gut to toxins such as endotoxins and peptidoglycan, causing inflammation and an immune response. Drinking alcohol can also activate pathogenic (gram-negative) bacteria to overgrow because alcohol feeds the bacteria. Alcohol can sometimes be tolerated in small quantities, around five ounces a week, despite these concerns, as long as you stay away from grain-based alcohol and white wine, which can produce yeast that acts as a cross-reactor of gluten.

Beans and Legumes

Beans and legumes, as they contain elevated amounts of saponins and protease inhibitors, are very similar to pseudograins. Increased intestinal permeability is linked to saponins and protease inhibitors. Legumes can have lectins, which may lead to leaky intestines as well.

Dairy Products

There are many explanations why people with autoimmune disease and even people without any health conditions may be affected by dairy products. Milk has lactose, a sugar that about 25 percent of people in the world can not tolerate in their systems. The hormone levels in the body can be changed by milk because it contains active bovine hormones. For an efficient immune system, hormone regulation is important. Dairy can lead to leaky intestines because it aids inflammation and includes protease inhibitors. Eating dairy can also boost mucus production, creating issues with the absorption of nutrients in the gut.

Avoid anything with dairy in it.

Eggs

While on the Autoimmune Paleo Diet, the whole egg is to be removed, although it is the egg white that generally triggers the problem rather than the yolk. There are no problems with yolks in certain persons with an autoimmune disease. The protective zone around the forming yolk is the egg whites. Egg whites contain antimicrobial proteins, and in people who have leaky intestines, these proteins may cause a negative reaction. The absorption of biotin (a B vitamin) can be interfered with by one of the proteins in egg whites, and another protein in whites inhibits the absorption of the protein itself. A worse problem with egg whites is that some of the compounds in them can pass through the barrier of the gut and cause additional damage as well as an immune response.

Stop all eggs, including baked goods, and everything made with eggs.

Grains

Plants have natural defensive mechanisms designed to avoid predators from eating them, humans are included amongst these predators. A class of proteins called lectins forms part of this defense mechanism. Digestive enzymes present in humans can not break down the structure of lectins, and because lectins contain protease inhibitors (enzymes that hinder protein breakdown), the digestive process is further impeded. This absence of digestion suggests that the lectins pass through the digestive system somewhat intact. Lectins are then transferred through the intestinal absorptive cells (enterocytes) that line the intestine by fooling the cells into believing that they are simple sugars. They cause an inflammatory response as the lectins move out of the gut, and this can damage or destroy the enterocyte, inhibiting healthy digestion and causing a leaky gut.

Most grains contain lectins, perhaps the best known of which is gluten. Since its composition is so similar to other proteins in the body, it can do an enormous amount of damage to the body. This implies that the regular cells of the body will also be targeted by at least a few of the antibodies produced to target gluten. Such antibody attacks are part of the mechanism that causes an autoimmune disorder and increases its intensity.

NSAIDs

NSAIDs are a source of gut discomfort and can exacerbate leaky intestines. However, it should be a personal choice to remove NSAIDs, since many autoimmune disorders are marked by excruciating pain that needs to be resolved. Pain is a traumatic experience, and healthy sleep habits can be totally disrupted by chronic pain. Stress and lack of sleep can make autoimmune disorders dramatically worse, but in the long run, treating pain with NSAIDs could facilitate healing. Discuss the choices with your doctor to make the healthiest decision for you if you need to treat pain associated with your autoimmune disorder.

Oils from Vegetables and Grains

These products are processed using chemicals that leave toxic residues. They are also very rich in omega-6 fatty acids and polyunsaturated fats. Due to their polyunsaturated fat content, vegetable oils oxidize readily, and this produces free radicals. Inflammation in the body can be increased by free radicals and too much omega-6 fatty acid has been shown to cause inflammation too.

Processed Foods

Usually, processed foods are filled with ingredients that are not conducive to healing or are commonly recommended for good health. Processing removes nutrients from food and also adds additives that can impede essential vitamins and minerals from being absorbed. The body is harmed by preservatives, emulsifiers, thickeners, dyes, stabilizers, and antinutrients that are produced during processing. The digestion of protein and minerals such as calcium, copper and zinc is impeded by anti-nutrients such as D-amino acids, lysinoalanine, oxidized sulfur amino acids, and additives such as guar gum, cellulose gum, xanthan gum, and lecithin. In several studies, including one published in 1983 in the Journal of Nutrition, guar gum and an additive called carrageenan were related to an improvement in the severity of the leaky intestine.

Eliminate all foods that have been refined, including emulsifiers, thickeners, and food additives.

Pseudograins

The edible seeds of broadleaf plants are pseudograins; they resemble grains but are not from the same biological community. Rather high levels of compounds called saponins produce pseudograins. Saponins are intended to discourage insects and microbes from consuming the plant. Saponins interact with molecules of cholesterol present in the body's cell membranes, forming gaps in the membranes. The contents of the gut may leak out when these holes are produced in the enterocytes that line the gut. These holes also destroy enterocyte cells, and along with inflammation in the body, intestinal permeability increases. Saponins also pass through the holes formed in the enterocytes and create bloodstream problems by damaging the red blood cell membranes. In the body, this leakage causes more inflammation.

Pseudograins also contain protease inhibitors alongside saponins. This is another defense of plants that neutralizes the enzymes in the digestive tract so that the protein in the plant can not be broken down into smaller amino acids. In the digestive tract, ingestion of pseudograins prevents protein degradation, and this can cause more enzymes to be secreted by the body. An surplus of certain enzymes and a deficiency of others can be produced by this cycle. Trypsin is one enzyme that typically ends up in abundance, and this enzyme is especially efficient in breaking down cell-to-cell connections such as enterocytes. An excess of trypsin can lead to intestinal leakage.

Seeds, Seed Oils, and Spices from Seeds

In certain people, seeds can increase inflammation, but they are one of the foods omitted from the Autoimmune Paleo Diet because they could cause problems, not because they certainly cause problems. Seeds are a source of lectin and phytic acid, both of which can enhance the permeability of the intestines and interfere with mineral absorption. Seeds are also rich in omega-6 fatty acids, which are capable of reducing the beneficial ratio of omega-3 to omega-6 fatty acids. Omega-6 fatty acids, meaning that they increase inflammation, are pro-inflammatory and omega-3 fatty acids are anti-inflammatory. A desirable ratio of these fatty acids ensures that more omega-3 than omega-6 fatty acids are absorbed, so that there is no inflammation in the net result.

Spices Made from Fruit

The spices derived from fruits are mostly mostly seeds, causing problems associated with the use of seeds. These spices are more on the list of 'proceed with caution' than the list of total exclusion, so it is a safe idea to exclude them from the Autoimmune Paleo Diet for at least the first 30 days.

Sweeteners, Sugar Alcohols, and Sugars

When you have an autoimmune disorder, sugar may cause many different problems, and refined sweeteners are especially damaging. Sugar, sweeteners, and alcohol with sugar can all irritate the gut and cause body tension. That's because minerals and vitamins are completely depleted in these processed sugar products. To metabolize the sugar, the body has to leech these nutrients from its own cells and tissues. This drain on the body is negative. Bacteria and yeast love to eat sugar, too, so it can induce overgrowth that leads to gut dysbiosis by including sweeteners in your diet.

FOODS TO EAT

You might be wondering what you will be eating now that you have seen the list of eliminated foods. You will be filling your plate with a colorful array of vegetables and fruits, organic meats and poultry, fresh fish and seafood, healthy fats, fragrant herbs, and fermented foods. There are so many tempting and delicious ingredients available to you that you will probably never get bored trying all of them.

MAIN COURSE

Honey ginger glazed salmon

Ingredient:

50ml of orange juice

50ml of honey

1 tbsp of olive oil

4 spring onions (Slice)

1 tbsp of fresh ginger(peeled)

1 tbsp of sherry vinegar

4 x 112g of salmon fillets

½ tsp of orange zest

Preparation:

1. Combine orange juice, spring onions, honey, olive oil, ginger, coconut aminos, sherry vinegar, and orange zest all together in a food processor. Allow it run for 30 seconds till it's completely combined.

2. Add marinade to a plastic bag with a ziplock. Add seal and salmon afterward you marinate and refrigerate salmon for an hour.

3. Set your medium-sized frypan to medium heat. Add salmon when the pan is hot with the skin side down. Put 50ml marinade over salmon and cook for 3 minutes.

4. Flip and cook till it's flaky and cooked through.

Recipe for 4 servings

Nutritional facts:

Calories: 249

Carbs: 22g

Fiber: 0g

Fat: 7g

Protein: 23g

Sunday Slow Cooker Pot Roast

Ingredient:

3-4 parsnips, chopped and peeled.

1 large-sized sweet potato peeled and chopped.

300g shallot, chopped

1.5kg boneless braising steak

2 tsp lemon juice

50ml of melted melted

350ml of beef stock

8 thinly sliced garlic cloves

1 ½ tsp of sea salt

1 tbsp tapioca starch

15g of chopped parsley

2 tbsp of Worcestershire Sauce

Preparation:

1. Put shallots, parsnips and sweet potatoes on a slow cooker.

2. Use a paring knife to make small cuts on both sides of the meat. Add garlic slices into these cuts and season it with meat and put 1 teaspoon sea salt.

3. Put the seasoned braising steak in a slow cooker, nestling it among the vegetables.

4. In a small bowl, whisk together beef stock, Worcestershire sauce, lemon juice and the remaining 1/2 teaspoon of sea salt. Pour the sauce over the meat in a slow cooker.

5. Cover and cook meat and vegetables in a slow cooker for 7 hours.

6. Remove the vegetables and meat with a slotted spoon from the slow cooker.

7. In a small bowl, whisk ghee, tapioca starch and parsley together. Add the contents to the juices in a slow cooker and stir to mix.

8. Slice the meat and spoon over the meat and vegetables with a slow-cooking sauce.

Recipe for 8 serving

Nutritional facts:

Calories: 369

Carbs: 23g

Fiber: 3g

Fat: 22g

Protein: 18g

Broccoli beef stir fry

Ingredients:

1 tbsp olive oil

½ large onion (chopped)

450g of thinly sliced skirt steak,

50ml of water

700g of chopped broccoli,

125ml of coconut aminos

125ml of beef stock

5 minced garlic cloves

1 tsp of fresh minced ginger

2 tbsp of fish sauce

1 tsp of honey

1 tsp of tapioca starch

Preparation:

1. Heat olive oil in a large pan over medium-high heat. Add onions and cook until soft and translucent.

2. Add the steak and cook for 5 minutes, turning regularly to brown on both sides.

3. Remove the steak and the onion from the frying pan and set aside. Add some water and broccoli.

4. Cover and steam 3 minutes until gentle. Take the broccoli out of the pan.

5. In a small cup, whisk together the coconut amino, beef stock, garlic, ginger, fish sauce, honey and tapioca starch.

6. Add the sauce to the frying pan and whisk over medium heat until it bubbles and starts to thicken. Return the meat and the broccoli to the pan and toss the coat.

Recipe for 4 servings

Nutrition:

Calories: 313

Carbs: 18g

Fiber: 3g

Fat: 16g

Protein: 24g

Greek-style roast chicken

Ingredients:

2.1kg roasting chicken,

without giblets Juice of 3 lemons

125ml of olive oil

¼ tsp of sea salt

¼ tsp of garlic powder

¼ tsp of onion powder

2 tbsp of dried oregano

10 cloves of minced garlic

1 large yellow onion (quartered)

2 medium sweet potatoes (cubed)

Preparation:

1. Preheat the oven to 190°C. Line the bottom of the baking bowl with parchment.

2. Rinse chicken with cold water and pat dry with kitchen towels. Using a sharp knife or a chicken shear, cut chicken in half along the spine. Remove the spine and put the two chicken halves on the baking parchment.

3. Pour the lemon juice over the chicken half, rubbing it in the flesh.

4. Drizzle the chicken with 50ml of olive oil and rub it into the chicken.

5. In a small cup, mix salt, garlic powder, onion and oregano.

6. Season chicken half with half the seasoning mixture.

7. In a big bowl, combine the garlic, the onion, the sweet potato, the remaining olive oil and the remaining half of the seasoning mixture. Toss in order to blend. Spread the onion and sweet potato mixture around the chicken portion.

8. Bake uncovered for 1 hour and 20 minutes, stirring regularly with juices from the bottom of the pan, holding the chicken moist.

Recipe for 8 servings

Nutrition:

Calories: 624

Carbs: 14g

Fiber: 3g

Fat: 41g

Protein: 51g

Apple Glazed Pork Chops

Ingredients:

350ml of unsweetened apple juice

50ml pure maple syrup

2 tbsp of Worcestershire Sauce

chops, bone in, with fat

1/8 tsp of cinnamon

4 x 110g of pork

1 tbsp olive oil

1 apple, cored and chopped

1/8 tsp sea salt

1 tsp fresh thyme, chopped

Preparation:

1. For apple glaze, mix apple juice, maple syrup, Worcestershire sauce and cinnamon in a small saucepan. Get the material to a boil. Reduce flame, cover and simmer for about 10 minutes. Remove the heat and set aside.

2. Heat olive oil in a skillet over medium-high heat. Season the pork chops with sea salt on both sides. Add pork chops and 125 ml apple glaze to the tip.

3. Cook pork chops for 5 minutes per side or until the internal temperature reaches 65°C, spoon sauce over pork chops periodically to avoid burning of the pan. Remove the pork chops from heat and set aside.

4. Add the chopped apple to the remaining saucepan. Get the content to a boil. Reduce heat and simmer for 10 minutes or until sauce has been reduced by at least half.

5. Place pork chops on a serving plate, top with apple and sauce mixture and garnish with fresh thyme.

Nutrients:

Calories: 300

Carbs: 31g

Fiber: 1g

Fat: 8g

Protein: 26g

Pork Tenderloin with Roasted Carrot Romesco

Ingredient:

680g of small

carrots, peeled and halved lengthwise

1⁄4 tsp sea salt

3 tbsp of olive oil

1 clove garlic (peeled)

450g of boneless pork tenderloin

2 tbsp of red wine vinegar

450g of rocket

Preparation:

1. Preheat the oven to 230°C. Line up a baking tray with foil.

2. Add 1 tablespoon of olive oil and 1⁄8 teaspoon of sea salt to the carrots. Place carrots on a baking tray and roast for 15 to 20 minutes, turning occasionally until tender. Remove the bread from the oven and set aside.

3. In a big, ovenproof pan, heat 1 tablespoon of olive oil over medium-high heat. Season the pork with 1⁄8 teaspoon of sea salt. Cook the

pork in the pan, stirring occasionally, for 10 to 15 minutes, until golden brown on all sides.

4. Move the pan to the oven and cook for another 8 to 10 minutes or until the tenderloin reaches 65ºC. Remove the pan from the oven, cover and let it sit for 5 minutes before cutting.

5. In a food processor, mix 1 tablespoon of olive oil, garlic, 1 tablespoon of red wine vinegar, 1 tablespoon of water and 1/3 of the toasted carrots. Process until it's smooth.

6. Place the rocket in a wide bowl with the remaining 1 tablespoon of red wine vinegar.

7. Arrange the remaining carrots and rocket on the serving tray. Cover with sliced pork tenderloin and drizzle with romesco carrot sauce.

Recipe for 4 servings

Nutrients:

Calories: 317

Carbs: 17g

Fiber: 5g

Fat: 17g

Protein: 25g

Meatfloaf muffins

Ingredients:

2 tbsp of olive oil

300g onion (chopped)

4 cloves garlic (minced)

2 celery stalks (chopped)

2 tbsp of coconut flour

2 tsp of Worcestershire Sauce

2 peeled and chopped carrots

1 tsp of dried oregano

1 tsp of marjoram

3 slices raw bacon (thinly sliced)

450g sweet potato (peeled and chopped)

1 tsp of dried basil

¾ tsp of sea salt

450g of minced beef

6g parsley (chopped)

2 tbsp of light coconut milk

1 tbsp of ghee

Preparation:

1. Preheat the oven to 190ºC. Heat olive oil in a large skillet over medium-high heat. Add onion, celery, carrots and 3 teaspoons of minced garlic. Cook for five minutes.

2. Add the marjoram, basil, oregano and 1⁄2 teaspoon of sea salt. Cook for 2 more minutes.

3. Move the vegetables to a wide bowl. Add beef, coconut flour, Worcestershire sauce and parsley to taste. Mix it to blend.

4. Spread the meat mixture over 12 cups of the muffin tin. Press the meat in a muffin tin and cover with 2 to 3 bits of bacon.

5. Bake meatloaf muffins for 20 minutes or until the internal temperature is 68°C.

6. To make the purée of sweet potatoes, cover the chopped sweet potatoes with water in a small saucepan. Get it to a boil. Reduce fire, cover and simmer for 10 minutes or until fork tender. Drain some sweet potatoes.

7. In a food processor, mix the sweet potatoes, coconut milk, 1 clove of garlic, the remaining 1⁄4 teaspoon of sea salt and ghee. Process for 30 seconds or until the process is smooth.

8. Cover meatloaf muffins with purée of sweet potatoes before serving.

Recipe for 6 servings

Nutrients:

Calories: 329

Carbs: 20g

Fiber: 5g

Fat: 21g

Protein: 17g

Blackened Chicken Breast

Ingredients:

450g boneless,

Skinless chicken breast

1½ tsp dried thyme

1 tsp coconut sugar

½ tsp Seed-Free

¼ tsp sea salt

1 tbsp olive oil

1½ tsp garlic powder

1½ tsp dried oregano

Curry Powder

Preparation:

1. Rinse chicken breasts under cold water and put in a large plastic zip lock bag. Using a meat tenderizer, pound meat into large, thin pieces.

2. Combine oregano, thyme, garlic powder, coconut sugar, seed-free curry powder and sea salt on a large plate. Toss to mix it up.

3. Coat chicken breasts with a combination of spices on both sides.

4. Heat olive oil in a large frying pan or grill pan over high heat.

5. Cook the seasoned chicken in olive oil for 3 to 5 minutes on each side until the chicken is finely blackened outside and cooked through.

6. Remove the chicken from the pan and let it sit for 5 minutes before it is sliced or served.

Recipe for 4 servings

Nutrients:

Calories: 164

Carbs: 3g

Fiber: 1g

Fat: 4g

Protein: 26g

Crispy Chicken Strips with Mango Honey Sauce

Ingredient:

450g boneless,

skinless chicken breast

2 tbsp of arrowroot powder

½ tsp of garlic powder

1 tbsp of honey

1 tbsp of cider vinegar

2 tbsp of coconut flour

1 spring onion (chopped)

1 clove of garlic (peeled)

125ml light coconut milk

60g of apricot preserves

Curry Powder

1 cup mango (peeled and chopped)

½ tsp of onion powder

1/4 tsp sea salt

60g of unsweetened shredded coconut

½ tsp Seed-Free

1 tbsp of lime juice

Preparation:

1. Pre-heat the oven to 200°C. Line up a baking tray with foil.

2. Rinse chicken breasts under cold water and put in a large plastic zip-lock container. Using a meat tenderizer, pound the meat in big, thin bits. Remove the chicken from the bag and cut it into 8 thin strips.

3. Combine coconut flour, arrowroot powder, garlic powder, onion powder and 1/8 tsp of sea salt on a large plate.

4. In a small cup, combine the coconut milk and the apricot mixture.

5. Combine shredded coconut and Seed-Free Curry Powder on a separate large dish.

6. Dry each chicken strip in a mixture of coconut flour, dip in a mixture of coconut milk and coat with a mixture of shredded coconut. Place the chicken strips on the prepared baking sheet.

7. Bake for about 15 minutes. Flip the chicken strips and bake for 15 minutes on the other side.

8. To make a dip sauce, combine the mango, spring onion, garlic, sugar, cider vinegar, lime juice and the remaining 1/8 tsp of sea salt in a food processor. Process until it's smooth.

Recipe for 4 servings

Nutrients

Calories: 376

Carbs: 39g

Fiber: 9g

Fat: 11g

Protein: 30g

Chimichurri Skirt Steak

Ingredients:

450g of skirt steak

1 tsp of sea salt

2 tbsp of dried oregano

½ shallot (peeled)

50g of parsley (loosely packed)

3 tbsp of sherry vinegar

3 tbsp of lemon juice

3 tbsp of olive oil

5 cloves garlic (peeled)

Preparation:

1. Remove the steak from the refrigerator and allow it to rise to room temperature.

2. In the meantime, mix parsley, sea salt, oregano, lemon juice, olive oil, sherry vinegar, garlic and shallot in a food processor. Process for 30 seconds or until the chimichurri has been well mixed.

3. Heat the pan over medium-high heat. Rinse steak, pat dry, and sprinkle with a pinch of salt on both sides.

4. Cook the steak on each side for 3 minutes, until it is sealed and brown.

5. Remove the steak from the plate, cover with foil and let it sit for 5 minutes before cutting.

6. Cut the steak in thin slices and top with chimichurri sauce.

Recipe for 4 servings

Nutrients:

Calories: 298

Carbs: 6g

Fiber: 2g

Fat: 20g

Protein: 25g

11 Burgundy Lamb Kebabs

Ingredients:

450g lamb stewing meat

1½ tbsp of dried parsley

2 tsp of olive oil

2 cloves of garlic (minced)

225ml of beef stock

¼ tsp of sea salt

225ml of red wine

½ tsp of lemon zest

Preparation:

1. Combine the lamb, garlic, parsley, olive oil, red wine, beef stock, sea salt and lemon zest in a big zip-lock container. Marinate for 8 to 10 hours or overnight.

2. Put 4 wooden skewers in a shallow water pan and soak for 30 minutes. Preheat barbecue to high heat.

3. Slice the onion into large bits. Remove the skewers from the bath.

4. Assemble the kebabs by threading the marinated bits of the lamb and the onions alternately on each skewer. Reserve an abundance of beef marinade.

5. Cook the skewers on the grill for 6 to 10 minutes, turn occasionally, and brush with a reserved marinade as required. Cook the lamb until the meat is 68ºC

Recipe for 4 servings

Nutrients:

Calories: 225

Carbs: 3g

Fiber: 0g

Fat: 8g

Protein: 24g

Triple-Berry Barbecued Ribs

Ingredients:

1½ racks of ribs (about 1.5kg total)

Barbecue Sauce

½ tsp sea salt

225ml of Triple-Berry

Preparation:

1. Cut each rack of ribs into smaller pieces and season with salt on both sides.

2. Brush the ribs liberally with barbecue sauce and put them in a slow cooker, piling them like shingles, one on top of the other.

3. Cook at the high temp for 7 hours. Meat ought to be tender and fall from the bones.

Recipe for 8 servings

Nutrients:

Calories: 465

Carbs: 11g

Fiber: 1g

Fat: 33g

Protein: 30g

Pineapple Teriyaki Salmon

Ingredient:

1 tbsp coconut oil

2 cloves garlic, minced

400g pineapple (chopped)

1 tbsp honey

½ tsp fish sauce

125ml coconut aminos

1 tsp of arrowroot powder

450g salmon, bones removed and skin on

Preparation:

1. Preheat the oven to 180°C.

2. Combine coconut oil and garlic in a small saucepan over medium-high heat. Stir and cook for 2 minutes or until fragrant.

3. Reduce heat to medium-low and add coconut amino, honey and fish sauce.

4. Gradually whisk in arrowroot powder until sauce is thickened. Remove the heat, cover and set aside.

5. Line up a baking dish with foil. Place the pineapple on the bottom of the pan. Place salmon on top of pineapple and a spoonful of sauce over the fish.

6. Bake for 15 minutes or until the fish is flaky and the pineapple soft and caramelized.

Recipe for 4 servings

Nutrients:

Calories: 221

Carbs: 15g

Fiber: 1g

Fat: 8g

Protein: 21g

Maple Balsamic Glazed Salmon

Ingredients:

450g salmon, skin

cut into 4 pieces

1/8 tsp of sea salt

50ml of balsamic vinegar

50ml of maple syrup

1 tbsp of olive oil

1 tbsp of molasses

2 cloves garlic (minced)

Preparation:

1. preheat the oven to 220°C

2. Line up a baking tray with foil. Put salmon on a baking sheet, skin-side down.

3. In a small bowl, mix maple syrup, balsamic vinegar, garlic, olive oil, molasses and salt.

4. Brush the salmon with the glaze, reserving any excesses. Bake for 5 minutes, brush with more glass and return to the oven. Repeat twice, baking salmon for a total of 15 minutes.

5. Enable salmon cool down on the tray for a few minutes before serving. Lift the flesh out of the skin to serve (the skin will stick to the foil). Dispose off the skin and the foil.

Recipe for 4 servings

Nutrients:

Calories: 245

Carbs: 20g

Fiber: 0g

Fat: 7g

Protein: 23g

Asian Turkey Lettuce Wraps

Ingredient:

10 prunes, pitted

2 tbsp red onion, diced

3 tbsp coconut aminos

1 tbsp honey

1⁄8 tsp sea salt

113g canned water (chestnuts, drained and chopped) 1½ tsp cider vinegar

3 cloves minced garlic

50g spring onions (chopped)

225ml water

450g minced turkey (preferably dark meat)

1 large onion (chopped)

1 tbsp of fresh ginger (peeled and minced)

16 large butterhead lettuce leaves (about 2 heads lettuce)

Preparation:

1. In a small saucepan ov

2. Bring contents to a boil, cover, and maintain low simmer. Simmer for 20 minutes later.

3. Take sauce off the heat and blend until smooth. Blend until smooth and set aside. Set aside. In a large frying pan over a medium-high heat, cook garlic, ginger, and onion. Mix in cooked turkey. Cook the meat for 5 to 10 minutes or until it turns brown and the onions are tender.

4. Add 2 tablespoons of water and half the plum sauce to the turkey mixture. Keep cooking for another five minutes.

5. After removing the pan from fire, stir in drained water chestnuts and spring onions.

6. Place one-quarter teaspoon of turkey meat mixture into each lettuce leaf. Drizzle in the remaining plum sauce.

Recipe for 4 servings

Nutrients:

Calories: 333

Carb: 32g

Fiber: 4g

Fat: 14g

Protein: 20g

Lemon Stuffed Sea Bass

Ingredient:

2 whole sea bass, cleaned

with gills and fins removed(about 1kg)

1 sliced lemon

4 sprigs rosemary

4 sprigs thyme

125ml dry white wine

4 sprigs parsley

2 tbsp of olive oil

2 cloves garlic, thinly sliced

1/8 tsp sea salt

Preparation:

1. Preheat the oven to 240°C.

2. Rub fish with a tablespoon of olive oil on all sides.

3. Arrange the fish cavity by installing half of the garlic slices, at least three lemon slices and at least two sprigs of rosemary, thyme and parsley.

4. Drizzle excess olive oil while the pan is still hot into the baking dish. Put fish on top. Pour half the wine over the fish in addition to salt and pepper to add flavor.

5. Bake for ten minutes. Prepare a baguette, pour the remaining white wine over the fish and bake until the fish flakes for another 10minutes.

6. Squeeze the lemon slices onto the fish before serving.

Recipe for 2 servings

Nutrients:

Calories: 333

Carb: 32g

Fiber: 4g

Fat: 14g

Protein: 20g

17 Bacon Wrapped Scallops

Ingredient:

450g of large

Sea scallops

50ml light coconut milk

2 tbsp of fresh coriander (chopped)

12 slices of bacon

Juice of 1 lime

Preparation:

1. Preheat grill. Line baking dish with aluminum foil.

2. Scallops should be rinsed under cold water, and then dried with paper.

3. Roll the scallop in a slice of bacon and secure it with a cocktail stick.

4. Put scallops on the cookie sheet and grilled for 6 minutes.

5. Cook for another 6 minutes in a hot skillet, turning until browned and cooked through.

6. Stir coconut milk, lime juice, and coriander together in a small cup.

7. A drizzle of coconut milk mixture over the scallops before serving.

Recipe for 4 servings

Nutrients:

Calories: 300

Carb: 7g

Fiber: 0g

Fat: 16g

Protein: 32g

Roast Duck with Shallots, Figs, and Honey

Ingredient:

2 x 225g duck breasts (skin on)

1/8 tsp of sea salt

3 tsp of fresh thyme (chopped)

2 tbsp of olive oil

150g dried figs (chopped and stems removed)

2 large leeks, white and green parts (thinly sliced)

125ml plus 1 tsp of red wine

4 carrots (peeled and chopped)

2 tbsp of honey

55g pancetta (chopped)

125ml vegetable stock

Preparation:

1. Set the oven to 180°C. Rinse duck meat under cold water and pat dry. To tenderize the duck breast, score the fat in a crisscross pattern. Season your duck breasts with salt and thyme.

2. In a big saucepan, melt olive oil over a medium-high flame. Add onions and carrots. Cook vegetables for 20 minutes or until they're tender.

3. Place duck breasts, skin side down, at the centre of the pan. Cook for ten minutes.

4. In a small bowl, mix honey and red wine and stir well. Brush breasts duck honey and turns.

5. Place in the oven and cook for ten minutes. Brush duck breasts in the honey mixture while continuing to roast the duck until internal temperature exceeds 74ºC .

6. In a frying pan, cook pancetta over a medium-high heat for 3 minutes or until crispy. Add dried figs, red wine, stock, and thyme to the pan. Stir contents as required, bring to a boil, reduce heat, and simmer for 10 minutes.

7. After removing the frying pan from the oven, let it sit for 5 minutes. Add fig sauce as topping before serving.

Recipe for 4 servings

Nutrients:

Calories: 577

Carb: 53g

Fiber: 7g

Fat: 25g

Protein: 37g

19 Orange Pulled Pork Carnitas

Ingredients:

1.6kg boneless pork shoulder

¼ tsp of sea salt

2 tbsp of olive oil

1 tbsp of dried oregano

Sliced (1 large onion)

1½ tsp of Seed-Free Curry Powder

300g red onion (thinly)

5 cloves garlic (sliced)

1 orange (halved)

Preparation:

1. Cook pork shoulder over low heat and let rest.

2. Stir together olive oil, salt, oregano, and Seed-Free Curry Powder in a small cup. Apply the mixture onto the pork shoulder.

3. Put pork shoulder in slow cooker. Add onions and garlic to the slow cooker, above the pork shoulder.

4. Squeeze the orange over the meat and vegetables and toss the remaining orange slices into the slow cooker. Cover and cook for eight hours on low.

5. Remove meat from the cooker and set it on the cutting board. Let the meat sit at room temperature for a while and use two forks to shred it.

Recipe for 6-7 servings

Nutrients:

Calories: 541

Carb: 4g

Fiber: 1g

Fat: 39g

Protein: 35g

Middle Eastern Bison Burgers

Ingredients:

450g minced bison

75gof chopped red onion (¼ large onion)

1 tbsp of olive oil

2 tsp of Seed-Free Curry Powder

5g of parsley (chopped)

2 cloves of garlic (minced)

1 tsp of salt

Preparation:

1. Combine minced bison, red onion, parsley, garlic, seed-free curry powder and salt in a wide cup.

2. In a bowl, blend ingredients together until well mixed and shape into 4 thick patties.

3. In a large frying pan over medium-high heat, heat olive oil. Add burger patties and cook, undisturbed for 4 minutes, without turning.

4. Flip burgers and continue cooking for 2 minutes on the other hand.

Recipe for 4 servings

Nutrients:

Calories: 291

Carb: 2g

Fiber: 0g

Fat: 22g

Protein: 22g

Herbed Baked Spaghetti Squash

Ingredients:

1 medium spaghetti squash (about 2kg)

1 tbsp of fresh thyme (chopped)

1 tbsp of fresh rosemary (chopped)

2 tbsp of olive oil

1/8 tsp of sea salt

Preparation:

1. Set the oven to 200ºC. Line a tray with foil.

2. Break the spaghetti squash lengthways. Scoop out and discard the seeds.

3. Put halves of squash on baking tray, flesh-side up. Cover each hand in olive oil, rubbing it into the flesh to ensure proper coat.

4. Infuse spices, including rosemary, thyme, and sea salt, into the squash halves.

5. Bake for approximately 30 to 45 minutes or until squash is fork tender.

6. After removing from the oven, allow it cool for 10 to 20 minutes. Using a fork, scoop the squash out of the skin before eating.

Recipe for 4 servings

Nutrients:

Calories: 100

Carb: 9g

Fiber: 2g

Fat: 8g

Protein: 1g

Garlic Pesto Courgette Pasta

Ingredients:

1 tbsp plus 175ml

olive oil

1 avocado, pit and skin removed

50g fresh basil leaves

1/8 tsp dried oregano

3 tbsp lemon juice

3 cloves garlic (peeled)

1/8 tsp dried thyme

Preparation:

1. In a medium sized frying pan, heat 1 tablespoon of olive oil over a medium-high heat. Add courgette noodles to the prepared pan and stir until slightly tender. Remove from the pan and set aside.

2. In a food processor mix remaining olive oil, garlic, oregano, thyme, basil, avocado, lemon juice, and sea salt. Process for thirty seconds or until smooth.

3. In a large bowl combine avocado pesto with courgette noodles.

Recipe for 8 servings

Nutrients:

Calories: 237

Carb: 5g

Fiber: 2g

Fat: 25g

Protein: 2g

Pad Thai Noodles

Ingredients:

4 medium carrots (peeled)

115g spring onions (chopped)

15g fresh coriander (chopped)

1 medium courgette (peeled)

2 tbsp of coconut oil

3 cloves of garlic (minced)

50ml fish sauce

2 tbsp coconut aminos

50ml lime juice

1 tbsp cider vinegar

255g broccoli slaw

1 lime, cut into wedges

Preparation:

1. Using a vegetable peeler, create long, thin slices using it across the vegetable.

2. In a large pan, mix coconut oil and garlic. Sauté the cabbage for two minutes or until soft.

3. Combine soy sauce, coconut aminos, lime juice, and apple cider vinegar. Simmer the sauce for 5 minutes or until you have reduced it by half.

4. Mix in carrots, broccoli slaw, courgette, and spring onions. Gently stir and grill for 2 to 3 minutes.

5. Remove pan from the heat and top with ground coriander and lime wedges.

Recipe for 3 servings

Nutrients:

Calories: 199

Carb: 17g

Fiber: 6g

Fat: 10g

Protein: 11g

Caramelized Plantain Porridge

Ingredients:

1 tablespoon coconut oil

2 cups coconut milk

2 ripe plantains, diced

1 teaspoon pure vanilla extract

¼ teaspoon ground ginger

1 tablespoon coconut sugar

¼ teaspoon ground turmeric

¼ cup unflavored collagen peptides (optional)

Preparation:

1. Melt the coconut oil in a big skillet over medium heat.

2. Add the plantains and cook for 5 minutes, stirring occasionally, so that they can caramelize and turn golden brown once the oil is hot.

3. Pour in the coconut milk, then add the vanilla, turmeric, and ginger to the mixture.

4. Bring the mixture to a boil, simmer and cover with a tight-fitting lid, then reduce the heat. For 5 minutes, simmer.

5. Remove the lid and, with a potato masher or large fork, gently mash the plantains. Put the lid back in and simmer for a further 5 minutes.

6. Remove the skillet from the heat and, just before serving, add the coconut sugar and collagen peptides (if used).

Recipe for 4 servings

Ingredients tips:

1. Make this dish your own by using a combination of spices. All the excellent additions to this dish are cinnamon, grated fresh ginger root, coconut flakes, and pure maple syrup.

2. In order to help heal the leaky gut, studies have shown that collagen is an important nutrient. At your local health food store or online, you can find collagen peptides.

Nutrients:

Calories: 440

Carb: 39g

Fiber: 5g

Fat: 32g

Protein: 6g

Bacon Date Spinach Sauté

12 ounces uncured bacon (diced)6 cups baby spinach (packed)

12 dates (pitted and diced)

2 cups riced cauliflower

1 teaspoon pure maple syrup

½ teaspoon salt

Preparation:

1. Place the diced bacon on the stovetop in a cold skillet. Turn the heat to medium-low and cook for 7 minutes, stirring occasionally, until the bacon begins to turn golden brown slightly.

2. Turn the heat off and drain approximately three-quarters of the fat from the pan carefully. Save the fat or discard it.

3. Over medium heat, return the pan to the stove, and add the dates and cauliflower rice. Cook, stirring frequently, for 2 minutes.

4. By the handful, add the packed spinach, letting it wilt before adding more to the pan. Stir for about 3 minutes, until all the spinach is wilted.

5. Turn the heat off; before serving, stir in the maple syrup and salt.

Recipe for 4 servings

Ingredient tip:

- In place of the spinach, you can use any type of dark leafy green. Try kale, Swiss chard, collard greens, or even turnip greens and switch things up.

- Pair this recipe with Hasselback Baked Sweet Potatoes for a big breakfast.

Nutrients:

Calories: 452

Carb: 25g

Fiber: 4g

Fat: 34g

Protein: 14g

SIDE DISH

Garlic Caper Roasted Cauliflower

Ingredient:

1 medium head cauliflower (cut into florets)

6g of fresh parsley (chopped)

2 tbsp of non-pareil capers (chopped)

1 tbsp of lemon zest

1 tbsp of coconut oil (melted)

2 tbsp of olive oil

50ml oflemon juice

1 clove of garlic (minced)

Preparation:

1. Set the oven to 200°C. Line baking pan with aluminum foil.

2. Spread cauliflower on baking sheet and drizzle with coconut oil, kneading the mixture into the florets to ensure they are well coated.

3. Roast the cauliflower for 15 minutes. Flip the cauliflower and roast until the edges are crisp and the pieces get golden brown.

4. In a small bowl, combine minced garlic, lemon zest, lemon juice, capers and olive oil. Whisk to mix.

5. Roasted cauliflower is tossed with dressing in a large bowl before serving.

Recipe for 2 servings

Nutrients:

Calories: 269

Carb: 19g

Fiber: 8g

Fat: 21g

Protein: 6g

Savoury Baked Butternut Squash

Ingredients:

1 butternut squash (sliced and seeds removed)

½ tsp of fresh rosemary (chopped)

1 tbsp of olive oil

½ tsp of fresh thyme (chopped)

Pinch of sea salt

Preparation:

1. Preheat the oven to 200°C. Line with foil a baking tray.

2. Place squash on the baking tray and drizzle with olive oil to ensure it is well coated by massaging it into the squash with clean hands.

3. Sprinkle the rosemary, thyme and sea salt with the squash.

4. For 10 minutes, roast squash. Flip and roast for another 10 minutes until the squash and fork-tender are golden brown.

Recipe for 4 servings

Nutrients:

Calories: 93

Carb: 16g

Fiber: 3g

Fat: 4g

Protein: 1g

Roasted Balsamic Green Beans

Ingredient:

450g green beans, vends trimmed and discarded

4 tsp of balsamic vinegar

1 tbsp of olive oil

Pinch of sea salt

Preparation:

1. Preheat the oven to 200°C. Line a foil-based baking tray.

2. Put the green beans on your baking tray. Add olive oil and 3 teaspoons of balsamic vinegar to the mixture.

3. With clean hands, massage the oil and vinegar into the green beans. Use sea salt to sprinkle.

4. For 10 minutes or until tender, roast green beans.

5. Remove the pan from the oven and add the remaining 1 teaspoon of balsamic vinegar to the green beans before serving.

Recipe for 4 servings

Nutrients:

Calories: 60

Carb: 6g

Fiber: 2g

Fat: 3g

Protein: 1g

Orange Cranberry Relish

Ingredients:

400g whole cranberries

75g sultanas

175ml maple syrup

1 tsp ground ginger

225ml water half an onion (chopped)

2 tsp ground cinnamon

1 medium apple (peeled and chopped)

225ml orange juice

Preparation:

1. Combine the cranberries, maple syrup, sultana, cinnamon, ginger, and water in a medium saucepan.

2. Heat for 15 minutes or until the cranberries have popped and begin to soften over medium-high heat, uncovered.

3. Add the orange juice, onion, and apple. Continue cooking, uncovered, until the mixture has thickened, for another 15 minutes.

Recipe for 9-10 servings

Nutrients:

Calories: 225

Carb: 58g

Fiber: 6g

Fat: 0g

Protein: 1g

Pan Seared Brussels Sprouts with Bacon

Ingredients:

4 slices bacon (chopped)

450g Brussels sprouts (trimmed and quartered)

Half of a large onion (chopped)

Preparation:

1. Cook the bacon in a large frying pan over medium-high heat for 5 minutes or until it is crisp.

2. To absorb excess grease, remove the bacon from the pan and place it on a clean plate lined with kitchen paper.

3. Cook the onion and the Brussels sprouts in the remaining bacon fat for 15 to 20 minutes or until tender and caramelized.

4. Remove the pan from the heat and mix the bacon into the mixture of Brussels sprouts.

Recipe for 6 servings

Nutrients:

Calories: 60

Carb: 7g

Fiber: 3g

Fat: 3g

Protein: 4g

Hasselback Sweet Potatoes

Ingredient:

4 medium sweet potatoes

4 garlic cloves (thinly sliced)

¼ tsp of salt

1 tbsp of fresh rosemary (finely chopped)

3 tbsp of ghee (melted)

1 tbsp of fresh sage (finely chopped)

Preparation:

1. Preheat the furnace to 190ºC.

2. Remove the potatoes and press each of the potato grooves with a piece of sliced garlic.

3. Place potatoes in a dish to bake. Sprinkle with rosemary, sage, and salt, and brush with melted ghee. Pan with foil cover.

4. Bake for 50 minutes or until you have fork-tender potatoes.

5. Before serving, remove the dish from the oven and spoon the juices from the bottom of the dish over the potatoes.

Recipe for 4 servings

Nutrients:

Calories: 194

Carb: 25g

Fiber: 4g

Fat: 10g

Protein: 3g

Cauliflower Fried Rice

Ingredient:

1 medium head cauliflower (cut into florets)

150g of onion (chopped)

150g of carrots (chopped)

1 tbsp of olive oil

1 clove of garlic (minced)

1 tbsp of Worcestershire Sauce

3 spring of onions (chopped)

1 tbsp of fresh ginger (peeled and minced)

1 tbsp of coconut aminos

Preparation:

1. Pulse the cauliflower in a food processor fitted with a chopping blade for 5 to 10 seconds or until it is finely grated and resembles rice.

2. Olive oil, onion, carrots, ginger, and garlic are added to a large frying pan over high heat. Cook until soft, or for 5 minutes.

3. Add the cauliflower, stir, and cook undisturbed for 5 minutes, allowing it to brown. Stir in the contents, scrape any browned bits from the bottom, and cook uninterrupted for another 5 minutes.

4. Simply remove the pan from the heat. Stir in coconut aminos, spring onions, and Worcestershire Sauce until the 'rice' is coated evenly.

Recipe for 4 servings

Nutrients:

Calories: 105

Carb: 17g

Fiber: 5g

Fat: 4g

Protein: 3g

Parsnip Purée

Ingredient:

300g (10½ oz) parsnips (peeled and chopped)

1 clove garlic (peeled)

2 tbsp of ghee

50ml of light coconut milk

¼ tsp smoked sea salt

Preparation:

1. Cover the parsnips and garlic in a medium saucepan with water. Over a high heat, cover and boil for 20 minutes.

2. Drain the parsnips, with the cooking liquid reserved.

3. Combine the cooked parsnips, garlic, ghee, coconut milk, and ghee in a food processor.

4. 50ml cooking liquid reserved, and sea salt smoked. 30 seconds or until smooth, process.

Recipe for 4 servings

Nutrients:

Calories: 234

Carb: 25g

Fiber: 6g

Fat: 15g

Protein: 2g

Coconut Butternut Squash Mash

Ingredient:

1 medium butternut squash, cut in half lengthways and seeds removed

2 tbsp plus 1 tsp maple syrup

3 tbsp of ghee

50ml light coconut milk

¼ tsp of sea salt

1⁄8 tsp of cinnamon

Preparation:

1. Preheat the oven to 190oC.

2. Line a baking tray with foil. Place the flesh-side-down butternut squash halves. Bake for 30 to 40 minutes or until tender with a fork.

3. Scoop out the skin of the butternut squash and put it in a food processor.

4. Ghee, coconut milk, maple syrup, and sea salt are added. 30 seconds or until smooth, process.

5. Scoop and sprinkle with cinnamon into a serving dish.

Recipe for 5 to 6 servings

Nutrients:

Calories: 124

Carb: 16g

Fiber: 3g

Fat: 7g

Protein: 1g

Roasted Tenderstem Broccoli with White Wine Mushrooms

Ingredient:

2 bunches tenderstem broccoli (leaves removed and ends trimmed)

1 tbsp of olive oil

1 tbsp of bacon fat

1 clove garlic (minced)

35g shallots (chopped)

225g cremini

50ml dry white wine

Preparation:

1. Preheat the oven to 200ºC. Line a foil-based baking tray.

2. On the baking sheet, place the tenderstem broccoli. Drizzle the vegetables with olive oil and massage the oil until well coated. For 10 minutes, roast.

3. Over medium-high heat, combine the bacon fat, shallots, garlic, mushrooms, and pancetta in a large frying pan. Sauté the vegetables for 10 minutes or until tender.

4. Deglaze the wine pan and allow the alcohol to cook for an additional 2 to 5 minutes.

5. Remove and transfer the tenderstem broccoli from the oven to a serving dish. Spoon over the tenderstem broccoli with white wine mushroom sauce.

Recipe for 4 servings

Nutrients:

Calories: 196

Carb: 10g

Fiber: 3g

Fat: 7g

Protein: 6g

Coriander Lime Vinaigrette

Ingredient:

1 clove garlic, peeled

1 tbsp fresh coriander (chopped)

3 tbsp lime juice

3 tbsp orange juice

50ml olive oil

1/8 tsp sea salt2 tbsp honey

1 tsp fresh ginger (peeled and minced)

Preparation:

1. Mix the garlic, lime juice, orange juice, honey, ginger, cilantro, olive oil, and sea salt together in a food processor.

2. 30 seconds or until smooth, process. Transfer to a container that is airtight.

Recipe for 1 serving

Nutrients:

Calories: 81

Carb: 6g

Fiber: 0g

Fat: 7g

Protein: 0g

Greek Red Wine Vinaigrette

Ingredient:

125ml of olive oil

2 tbsp of red wine vinegar

2 tbsp of lemon juice

1 tsp of dried oregano

1 clove garlic (peeled)

¼ tsp of sea salt

Preparation:

1. Mix the olive oil, lemon juice, red wine vinegar, garlic, oregano, and sea salt together in a food processor.

2. 30 seconds or until smooth, process. Transfer to a container that is airtight.

Recipe for 1 serving

Nutrient:

Calories: 163

Carb: 1g

Fiber: 0g

Fat: 18g

Protein: 0g

Strawberry Lemon Vinaigrette

Ingredient:

125ml olive oil

50ml orange juice

600g strawberries, hulled

2 cloves garlic (peeled)

1 tsp lemon zest

1 tbsp of lemon juice

1 tbsp of balsamic vinegar

1/8 tsp sea salt

Preparation:

1. Combine the strawberries, olive oil, orange juice, lemon juice, balsamic vinegar, garlic, lemon zest and sea salt in the food processor.

2. 30 seconds or until smooth, process. Transfer to a container that is airtight.

Recipe for 1 serving

Nutrient:

Calories: 73

Carb: 3g

Fiber: 1g

Fat: 7g

Protein: 0g

Carrot Ginger Dressing

Ingredient:

75g carrot (peeled and chopped)

125ml of water

1 tbsp of olive oil

3 tbsp of light coconut milk

2 tbsp of cider vinegar

2 tbsp of honey

2 tbsp of fresh ginger (minced)

1/8 tsp of sea salt

2 tbsp of lemon juice

Preparation:

1. Combine the carrots and water in a small saucepan. Just bring it to a boil. Reduce heat, cover and cook for 20 minutes or until tender.

2. Transfer the carrots and boiling water to the food processor and add the ginger, sea salt, cider vinegar, lemon juice, honey, coconut milk, and olive oil.

3. 30 seconds or until smooth, process. Transfer to a container that is airtight.

Recipe for 1 serving

Nutrient:

Calories: 20

Carb: 3g

Fiber: 1g

Fat: 7g

Protein: 0g

Apple Currant Celeriac Slaw

Ingredient:

1 large bulb celeriac (peeled and quartered)

1½ large apples (peeled and quartered)

Juice and zest of 1 lemon

1/8 tsp of sea salt

1 tbsp of orange juice

1 tbsp of fresh thyme (chopped)

2 tbsp of fresh basil (chopped)

75g dried currants, or raisins

Preparation:

1. Fit the food processor with a disc shredding attachment. Feed the apple and celeriac quarters into the grating machine.

2. Combine the orange juice, lemon juice, lemon zest, and salt in a small bowl to make the dressing.

3. Combine the grated celeriac and apple mixture with thyme, basil, and currants in a large bowl.

4. To combine, pour dressing over slaw and toss. Before serving, let it sit for 5 minutes.

Recipe for 4 serving

Nutrient:

Calories: 171

Carb: 42g

Fiber: 6g

Fat: 0g

Protein: 3g

Mediterranean Tuna Salad

Ingredient:

4 x 170g cans albacore tuna (drained)

1 x 395g can artichoke hearts (drained and chopped)

50g of celery (chopped)

1 tsp of dried oregano

115g Basic Avocado "Mayonnaise"

150g of red onion (chopped)

6g parsley (chopped)

75g of cucumber (chopped)

140g of green olives (pitted and chopped)

6g fresh basil (chopped)

½ tsp of sea salt

Preparation:

1. 1 Combine the tuna, artichoke hearts, celery, cucumber, green olives, red onion, parsley, basil, oregano, Mayonnaise Basic Avocado, and sea salt in a large bowl. Stir gently until mixed well.

2. 2 Before serving, refrigerate the salad for 15 minutes to allow the flavours to come together.

Recipe for 8 servings

Nutrient:

Calories: 192

Carb: 6g

Fiber: 3g

Fat: 10g

Protein: 18g

Avocado Chicken Salad

Ingredient:

560g cooked chicken
breast, chopped

150g red onion (finely chopped)

150g cucumber (finely chopped)

1 clove garlic, minced Juice of 1½ limes

½ tsp sea salt

15g fresh coriander (chopped)

2 avocados (mashed)

Preparation:

1. Combine the chicken, cucumber, red onion, garlic, lime juice, fresh cilantro, mashed avocado and sea salt in a large mixing bowl. Stir gently until mixed well.

2. Before serving, refrigerate the salad for 30 minutes to allow the flavours to come together.

Recipe for 6 servings

Nutrient:

Calories: 283

Carb: 7g

Fiber: 3g

Fat: 10g

Protein: 18g

Shaved Broccoli and Cauliflower Slaw

Ingredients:

1.4kg of broccoli florets

600g of cauliflower florets

125ml lemon juice

125ml pineapple juice

375g carrots (peeled and roughly chopped)

25g of parsley (chopped)

300g of raisins

1 tbsp of lemon zest

¼ tsp of sea salt

Preparation:

1. Fit a shredding disk attachment to the food processor. Feed the machine with broccoli and pulse until thinly shredded. Transfer to a spacious bowl.

2. Feed the cauliflower to the food processor for grating. Transfer the broccoli to a large bowl.

3. Feed the carrots into the food processor, pulse until they are finely shredded, and add the broccoli and cauliflower to the bowl. Stir to mix.

4. To the vegetable mixture, add raisins and parsley and stir to combine.

5. Whisk the lemon juice, pineapple juice, lemon zest, and salt together in a small bowl. To combine, pour dressing over slaw and toss.

6. To allow the flavours to come together, refrigerate for 20 minutes before serving.

Recipe for 6 to 7 servings

Nutrient:

Calories: 274

Carb: 67g

Fiber: 9g

Fat: 1g

Protein: 8g

Citrus Mint Salad

Ingredients:

2 oranges (peeled and sliced)

1 grapefruit (peeled and sliced)

1 tbsp of fresh mint leaves (chopped)

2 tbsp of lime juice

2 tbsp of honey

180g if pomegranate seeds

Preparation:

1. Arrange the orange, grapefruit and pomegranate seeds on a large platter.

2. Whisk the lime juice and honey together in a small bowl.

3. Sprinkle with fruit dressing and garnish with mint leaves.

Recipe for 4 servings

Nutrient:

Calories: 133

Carb: 33g

Fiber: 4g

Fat: 1g

Protein: 2g

Honey Vinegar Tri-Coloured Coleslaw

Ingredients:

300g of red cabbage (shredded)

2 carrots (peeled and shredded)

300g green cabbage (shredded)

2 tbsp of cider vinegar

4 tbsp of olive oil

2 tbsp of honey

¼ tsp of sea salt

50g spring onions (chopped)

1 clove garlic (minced)

15g fresh coriander (chopped)

Preparation:

1. Combine the red cabbage, green cabbage, carrots, and spring onions in a large bowl.

2. Whisk the cider vinegar, olive oil, garlic, honey, and sea salt together in a small bowl.

3. Pour the dressing over the mixture of cabbage and toss to cover. Stir the fresh cilantro in.

4. Refrigerate before serving for 5 to 10 minutes to allow the flavours to come together.

Recipe for 9 servings

Nutrient:

Calories: 109

Carb: 12g

Fiber: 3g

Fat: 6g

Protein: 1g

Classic Kale Salad

Ingredients:

400g (14oz) butternut squash (peeled and cubed)

1 tbsp of olive oil

2 tbsp of lemon juice

1/8 tsp of sea salt

30g of dried cranberries

550g kale, stems removed and roughly chopped

2 tbsp of Greek Red Wine Vinaigrette

1 tbsp of honey

Preparation:

1. 1 Preheat the oven to 190°C.

2. Line a baking tray with foil. On a baking tray, spread the butternut squash, drizzle with the olive oil and sprinkle with sea salt. For 10 minutes, bake.

3. Combine the kale, lemon juice, and Greek Red Wine Vinaigrette in a large bowl while the squash bakes. Massage the dressing into kale leaves with clean hands.

4. Pull the squash out of the oven. Turn the pieces over and bake for an additional 5 minutes.

5. Drizzle with honey, remove the squash from the oven, and bake for another 5 minutes.

6. Add the kale to the squash and dried cranberries and toss until mixed.

Recipe for 2 servings

Nutrient

Calories: 218

Carb: 35g

Fiber: 5g

Fat: 9g

Protein: 5g

Asian Cucumber Salad

Ingredients:

2 medium cucumbers, sliced into (6mm) ¼-inch slices

1 tsp sea salt

1 tbsp of sherry vinegar

1 tbsp of honey

1 tbsp of white wine vinegar

40g of red onion (thinly sliced)

Preparation:

1. Use a bowl or sink to put cucumber slices into a colander. Sprinkle with salt from the sea and leave to drain for 30 minutes.

2. Use kitchen paper or a clean dish towel to remove cucumber slices from the colander and squeeze out the excess water.

3. Combine the cucumber and red onion in a large bowl.

4. Whisk together the honey, white wine vinegar and sherry vinegar in a small bowl.

5. Pour over the cucumber salad dressing and toss to combine.

Recipe for 2 servings

Nutrient:

Calories: 84

Carb: 21g

Fiber: 2g

Fat: 0g

Protein: 2g

Grilled Chicken Cobb Salad

Ingredients:

3 x 170g boneless (skinless chicken breasts)

1 tbsp olive oil

600g romaine lettuce (chopped)

1 large avocado (chopped)

1/4 tsp sea salt

300g cucumber (peeled and chopped)

115g spring onions (chopped)

15g parsley (chopped)

6 slices bacon (cooked and chopped

Preparation:

1. Place your chicken breasts between two sheets of parchment for baking. Punch to an even thickness of 1.25cm (1⁄2 inch) with a meat tenderizer.

2. Brush the chicken breasts with olive oil on both sides and season with sea salt.

3. Heat a medium-high grill. Place the chicken breasts on the grill and cook for about 3 to 5 minutes, until the bottom is browned. Flip and cook until cooked, about 3 to 5 more minutes.

4. Set aside to cool and remove the chicken from the grill. Chop into bite-size pieces when cool enough to touch.
5. On each salad plate, place the romaine lettuce. Work in rows with avocado, parsley, bacon, cucumber, spring onions, and chicken top lettuce.

Recipe for 4 servings

Nutrient:

Calories: 325

Carb: 12g

Fiber: 7g

Fat: 20g

Protein: 28g

Caribbean Chicken Salad

Ingredient:

3 x 170g of boneless/Skinless chicken breasts

¼ tsp of sea salt

300g mixed greens

1 tbsp of olive oil

1 mango (peeled and sliced)

15g unsweetened (shredded coconut)

30g of dried cranberries

1 cucumber (peeled and sliced)

1 jicama (or crisp green apple), peeled and chopped

115g of spring onions (sliced)

Preparation:

1. Place your chicken breasts between two sheets of parchment for baking. Punch to an even thickness of 1.25cm (1⁄2 inch) with a meat tenderizer.

2. Brush the chicken breasts with olive oil on both sides and season with sea salt.

3. The Medium-High Heat Grill. Place the chicken breasts under the grill and cook for about 3 to 5 minutes, until the bottom is browned. Turnover and cook for about 3 to 5 minutes more, until cooked through.

4. Remove the grilled chicken and let it cool. Slice into strips when cool enough to touch.

5. Toss the mixed greens, jicama, mango, cucumber, and spring onions into a large bowl to combine.

6. Sliced chicken salad, shredded coconut, and cranberries.

Recipe for 4 servings

Nutrient:

Calories: 303

Carb: 36g

Fiber: 12g

Fat: 8g

Protein: 25g

DESSERT

Sea Salt Caramel Sauce

Ingredients:

50ml of cup coconut cream

2 tbsp of coconut sugar

50ml of honey

Dash sea salt

1 tbsp of vanilla extract

1 tbsp ghee

Preparation:

1. Bring your coconut cream, honey, and coconut sugar to a boil in a small saucepan over medium heat.
2. Add the vanilla and sea salt extract and reduce the heat to low.
3. Simmer for 5 minutes, frequently stirring.
4. Remove from heat and stir until melted and combined, adding ghee.

Recipe for 1 serving

Nutrient:

Calories: 78

Carb: 12g

Fiber: 0g

Fat: 3g

Protein: 0g

51 Coconut Whipped Cream

Ingredients:

1 x 400ml can of full-fat coconut milk

3 tbsp of maple syrup

50ml coconut water

Preparation:

1. In your fridge, put the can of full-fat coconut milk and chill overnight.
2. Chill in the freezer with a metal mixing bowl for 5 minutes.
3. Scoop out the can of coconut cream into the chilled bowl, leaving behind the coconut water that has settled down to the bottom of the can.
4. Whip coconut cream with a low to creamy electric mixer (about 1 minute).
5. Add coconut water and maple syrup and, until light and fluffy, continue whipping (about 2 minutes).

Recipe for 7 servings

Nutrient:

Calories: 146

Carb: 9g

Fiber: 0g

Fat: 12g

Protein: 0g

Orange Cream Ice Lolly

Ingredients:

1 x 400ml can light coconut milk

225ml freshly squeezed orange juice

1 tbsp of orange zest

4 tbsp maple syrup

Preparation:

1. Whisk together the coconut milk and 2 tablespoons of maple syrup in a large bowl until smooth.
2. Pour the coconut mixture into a mould of ice lolly, halfway filling each mould. 10 minutes to freeze.
3. Whisk together the orange juice, orange zest, and the remaining 2 tablespoons of maple syrup in a small bowl.
4. Remove the mixture of coconut from the freezer, add the mixture of orange juice to the moulds, and insert the sticks. Freeze for 12 to 24 hours or until thoroughly frozen.

Recipe for 12 servings

Nutrient:

Calories: 47

Carb: 7g

Fiber: 0g

Fat: 2g

Protein: 0g

Warm Cinnamon Apples

Ingredients:

1 tbsp ghee

1 tsp of vanilla extract

2 medium apples (peeled and chopped)

2 tbsp maple syrup

75g raisins

1⁄4 tsp cinnamon

Preparation:

1. Heat ghee over medium heat in a big frying pan.
2. Add apples, raisins, maple syrup, cinnamon, and vanilla extract. Stir to mix.
3. Cover and cook for 20 minutes or until you have fork-tender apples.
   Recipe for 4 servings

Nutrient:

Calories: 168

Carb: 36g

Fiber: 3g

Fat: 4g

Protein: 1g

Honey Fried Bananas

Ingredients:

125ml of warm water

2 tbsp of coconut oil

1 tbsp of honey

2 medium under ripe bananas (peeled and sliced)

1/8 tsp cinnamon

Preparation:

1. Whisk the warm water and honey together in a small bowl.
2. Heat the coconut oil over medium to high heat in a large frying pan.
3. Add slices of banana and fry for 2 minutes. Flip and fry for another 2 minutes or until the bananas on both sides are a crisp golden brown.
4. Remove the pan from the heat and pour the mixture of honey and water over the bananas.
5. Before serving, sprinkle with cinnamon and let cool slightly.

Recipe for 4 servings

Nutrient:

Calories: 127

Carb: 18g

Fiber: 2g

Fat: 7g

Protein: 1g

Caramel Coconut Macaroons

Ingredients:

90g of unsweetened

Shredded coconut

2 tbsp of coconut flour

2 tbsp of coconut oil

1 tbsp of vanilla extract

50ml of Sea Salt

50ml of maple syrup

1⁄4 tsp of sea salt

Caramel Sauce

Preparation:

1. Preheat the heat to 180ºC in the oven. Line a baking tray with parchment for baking.
2. Combine the shredded coconut, coconut oil, coconut flour, vanilla extract, maple syrup and sea salt in a food processor. Process for 30 seconds or until the ingredients have the texture of wet sand and are well combined.
3. Scoop the batter into 1-tablespoon portions on the baking tray.
4. For 10 minutes, bake. Rotate the pan and cook for 5 more minutes or until the pan is golden brown.
5. Before transferring to the wire rack, let the pan cool for 5 to 10 minutes. Drizzle with Sea Salt Caramel Sauce when totally cool.

Recipe for 16 servings

Nutrient:

Calories: 59

Carb: 5g

Fiber: 1g

Fat: 4g

Protein: 1g

Avocado Pineapple Smoothie

Ingredients:

75g of kale (chopped and tightly packed)

225ml of orange juice

50g avocado (chopped 4-5 ice cubes)

115g pineapple (roughly chopped

Preparation:

1. Combine the kale, orange juice, pineapple, avocado, and ice cubes in a blender.
2. Blend until smooth, or for 30 seconds.

Nutrient:

Calories: 218

Carb: 34g

Fiber: 6g

Fat: 9g

Protein: 5g

Creamy Coconut Milk Hot Cocoa

Ingredients:

450ml of light coconut milk

2 tbsp of maple syrup

2 tbsp of carob powder

1 tsp of vanilla extract

1⁄2 tsp of cinnamon

50ml of water

Preparation:

1. Whisk the coconut milk, carob powder, maple syrup, vanilla extract, cinnamon and water together in a small saucepan over low heat.
2. Heat for 5 minutes, while stirring until the contents are warm and mixed.

Recipe for 2 servings

Nutrient:

Calories: 241

Carb: 39g

Fiber: 9g

Fat: 12g

Protein: 1g

Blueberry Lemon Cheesecake

Ingredients:

3 cups of dates, pitted and soaked for 5 minutes in warm water

1 cup of coconut oil (melted)

1/3 cup of coconut flour

1/3 of cup shredded coconut

1/8 of teaspoon salt

1 cup of raw honey (softened)

3/4 cup of coconut oil (softened)

1 cup of coconut cream (softened)

fresh blueberries for garnish

3 cups of frozen blueberries

1 lemon, juice and zested

1/8 of teaspoon salt

4 tablespoons of tapioca starch

1 teaspoon of vanilla extract

Preparation:

1. To let them soften, place the jars of coconut oil, coconut butter and raw honey in a pan with very hot water.
2. Preheat your oven to 325 degrees to prepare the crust. Strain the dates and place them with the melted coconut oil in a food processor or high-powered blender. Blend until a chunky paste forms, for 30 seconds or so. Be warned that if you are using a blender, you may have to stop and scrape the sides and the oil may not mix completely with the dates, but the crust will still turn out fine.
3. In a bowl, mix the coconut flour, shredded coconut and salt together. Add and thoroughly mix the date paste. Using your fingers to push it up and form it evenly around the sides, place the mixture into the bottom of a pie dish. Bake for 30-35 minutes, until the crust is slightly brown and hard. Until it completes cooling, the texture will still be soft. While you make the filling, set aside.

4. Combine the raw honey, coconut butter, coconut oil, and frozen blueberries in a low-heat saucepan to make the filling. Stir for about 5 minutes until the berries are no longer frozen and the mixture is warm. Put the tapioca starch, vanilla extract, lemon juice, zest, and salt in a blender. Blend for about a minute on high, until mixed completely. On top of the crust, pour carefully into the springform pan.

5. To allow the cake to cool and completely harden, set in the refrigerator undisturbed for at least 12 hours.

6. Decorate the top of the cake with fresh blueberries when it is solid.

Recipe for 8 servings

Nutrient:

Calories: 327

Carb: 27g

Fiber: 1g

Fat: 23g

Protein: 4g

Raspberry Coconut Cheesecake

Ingredients:

1 cup of coconut oil, melted

1/3 cup of shredded coconut

1/3 cup of coconut flour

1/8 teaspoon of salt

1½ cups of raw honey, softened

1 cup of coconut oil, softened

5 cups of frozen raspberries

1½ cups of coconut cream, softened

1½ teaspoons of vanilla extract (optional)

6 tablespoons of tapioca starch

1/4 teaspoon of salt

fresh raspberries for garnish

thick coconut flakes for garnish

Preparation:

1. To let them soften, place the jars of coconut oil, coconut butter and raw honey in a pan with very hot water.
2. Preheat your oven to 325 degrees to prepare the crust. Strain the dates and place them with the melted coconut oil in a food processor or high-powered blender. Blend until a chunky paste forms, for 30 seconds or so. Be warned that if you use a blender, you may have to stop and scrape the sides and the oil may not mix completely with the dates, but the crust will still turn out fine.
3. In a bowl, mix the coconut flour, shredded coconut and salt together. Add and thoroughly mix the date paste. In an 8-inch spring-form pan, place the mixture on the bottom, pressing it down evenly.
4. To clean up the upper edge around the sides of the pan, use a small spatula where the filling meets the crust. Bake for 30-35 minutes, until the crust is a little bit brown and hard. Until it completes cooling, the texture will still be soft. While you make the filling, set aside.

5. Combine the raw honey, coconut butter, coconut oil, and frozen raspberries in a low-heat saucepan to make the filling. Stir for about 5 minutes, until the raspberries are no longer frozen and the mixture is warm. Transfer the tapioca starch, vanilla extract, and salt to a blender. Blend for about a minute on high, until mixed completely. On top of the crust, pour carefully into the spring-form pan.

6. To allow the cake to cool and completely harden, set in the refrigerator undisturbed for at least 12 hours. Carefully remove the spring-form pan when it is solid.

7. Decorate the top of the cake with fresh raspberries and thick coconut flake chips.

Recipe for 12 servings

Nutrient:

Calories: 160

Carb: 32g

Fiber: 0g

Fat: 8g

Protein: 1g

Blueberry Macaroons

Ingredients:

2 cups of fine coconut flakes

1 cup of blueberries, frozen

1 cup of dates (pitted and soaked in warm water for 5 minutes)

¼ teaspoon of sea salt

¼ teaspoon of alcohol-free vanilla extract (optional)

2 tablespoons of fine coconut flakes

Preparation:

1. Preheat your oven up to 325 degrees.
2. In a food processor, place the coconut flakes, dates, blueberries, vanilla, and sea salt and process them until thick and sticky.
3. Shape into small balls, roll with coconut flakes for decoration.
4. Place on a greased sheet of cookies and cook for 12-15 minutes or until barely golden.

Recipe for 12 servings

Nutrient:

Calories: 60

Carb: 8g

Fiber: 1g

Fat: 3g

Protein: 2g

Apple cinnamon bars

Ingredients:

3 cups fine coconut flakes

¼ teaspoon sea salt

2 cups dried apple rings

¼ cup coconut oil

½ cup dates, pitted and soaked in warm water for 5 minutes

2 teaspoons cinnamon

Preparation:

1. Preheat up to 325 degrees in your oven.
2. In a food processor, place the coconut flakes, apple rings, dates, coconut oil, cinnamon, and sea salt and process them until they are thick and sticky.
3. Press firmly into an 8x8 baking pan that is greased. Bake until golden, or 25 minutes.
4. Score in bars whilst still warm. To harden, let it cool and refrigerate.
Recipe for 4 servings

Nutrients:

Calories: 200

Carb: 24g

Fiber: 1g

Fat: 7g

Protein: 10g

Apple-Spice Tea cookies

Ingredients:

3 cups of fine coconut flakes

2 cups of dried apple rings

¼ cup of coconut oil

½ cup of dates, pitted and soaked in warm water for 5 minutes

¼ teaspoon of sea salt

2 teaspoons of cinnamon

Preparation:

1. Preheat your oven up to 325 degrees.
2. In a food processor, place the coconut flakes, apple rings, dates, coconut oil, cinnamon, and sea salt and process them until they are thick and sticky.
3. Press firmly into an 8x8 baking pan that is greased. Bake until golden, or 25 minutes.
4. Score in bars whilst still warm. To harden, let it cool and refrigerate.

Recipe for 8 servings

Nutrients:

Calories: 120

Carb: 21g

Fiber: 1g

Fat: 4g

Protein: 2g

Cinnamon Tapioca Pudding

You might have fond memories of tapioca pudding from your childhood, but you may have never known that tapioca is actually derived from the cassava tuber, which appears often in this book in its flour form. Cassava flour is naturally allergen-friendly, making it an ideal option for those following the autoimmune protocol. Although desserts and sweet treats should be enjoyed in moderation to minimize blood sugar spikes, it's nice to have a sweet and comforting dessert option on hand. MAKES 4 SERVINGS

Preparation:

Prep time: 5 minutes

Cook time: 25 minutes

3 tablespoons quick-cooking tapioca

⅓ cup coconut sugar

2 tablespoons unflavored collagen peptides

1 teaspoon ground cinnamon

2 (14-ounce) cans light coconut milk

1 teaspoon pure vanilla extract

⅛ teaspoon salt

1.In a medium saucepan, combine the tapioca, coconut sugar, collagen peptides, cinnamon, and coconut milk. Stir well and let stand for 5 minutes.

2.Place the pan over medium heat. Bring the mixture to a boil, stirring constantly. Boil for 1 minute, then turn off the heat and stir in the vanilla and salt.

3.Allow to stand for 20 minutes before serving warm or chilled.

Nutrients:

Calories: 80g

Carb: 24g

Fiber: 3g

Fat: 4g

Protein: 2g

DRINKS (JUICE/SMOOTHIES)

Anti inflammatory matcha latte

Ingredients:

2 tablespoons of unflavored collagen peptides (optional)

¼ cup of filtered water

2 teaspoons of pure matcha powder

½ teaspoon of ground ginger

2 cups of light coconut milk

1 tablespoon of coconut sugar

½ teaspoon of pure vanilla extract

Preparation:

1. Bring the water to a boil in a medium saucepan over a medium-high heat. To form a paste, turn off the heat and whisk in the matcha powder.
2. Return the heat to low and stir in the coconut milk, coconut sugar, and ginger. Cook on low heat, stirring occasionally, for 5 minutes, or until ready to boil.
3. Stir in the vanilla extract and collagen peptides just prior to serving (if using).

Recipe for 2 servings

Ingredient tips

- Although the collagen peptides in this recipe are optional, it is strongly recommended that you add them whenever possible for their nutritional value. Each tablespoon of collagen peptides provides 10 grams of high-quality protein that can help the gut heal after your morning meal and keep you full and satisfied.

Nutrients:

Calories: 164

Carb: 16g

Fiber: 1g

Fat: 12g

Protein: 4g

Mango Turmeric Lassi

Ingredients:

1 cup of diced frozen mango

1 cup of filtered water

1 tablespoon of pure maple syrup

1 cup of sliced frozen carrots

1 cup of Creamy Coconut Milk Yogurt

½ teaspoon of ground turmeric

2 tablespoons unflavored collagen peptides (optional)

Preparation:

1. Add the mango, carrots, yogurt, coconut milk, water, maple syrup, turmeric, and collagen peptides to the blender (if using).
2. Blend for two minutes on high, or until completely smooth.

Recipe for 2 servings

Ingredients tips:

- As long as there are no other added ingredients, frozen fruits and vegetables are just as nutritious as fresh. Buying frozen fruit helps reduce preparation time, can save you cash, and creates a cold, creamy consistency that's perfect for this drink.
- It is strongly recommended that you add them whenever you can for their nutritional value, although the collagen peptides are optional in this recipe. Each tablespoon of collagen peptides provides 10 grams of high-quality protein which, after your morning meal, can help the gut heal and keep you full and satisfied.

Nutrients:

Calories: 341

Carb: 36g

Fiber: 6g

Fat: 24g

Protein: 1g

Bright Green Detox Smoothie

Ingredients:

2 celery stalks (diced)

1 cup baby spinach (packed)

1 green apple (cored and diced)

1 avocado (pitted and scooped)

1 cup ice cubes

1 cup freshly squeezed orange juice or filtered water

1 small cucumber (diced)

½-inch piece peeled fresh ginger root

2 tablespoons unflavored collagen peptides (optional)

Preparation:

1. Add the celery, avocado, spinach, apple, cucumber, ginger, ice, orange juice and peptides of collagen to a blender (if using).
2. Blend for two minutes on high, or until completely smooth.

Recipe for 2 servings

Ingredient tips

- Green smoothies are so flexible, and it is possible to interchange the ingredients and still taste delicious. Try adding a frozen banana if you're struggling with the taste of a green smoothie. This will make it creamier and sweeter for the recipe.

- It is strongly recommended that you add them whenever you can for their nutritional value, although the collagen peptides are optional in this recipe. Each tablespoon of collagen peptides provides 10 grams of high-quality protein which, after your morning meal, can help the gut heal and keep you full and satisfied.

Nutrients:

Calories: 291

Carb: 43g

Fiber: 10g

Fat: 14g

Protein: 5g

Triple Berry Antioxidant Smoothie

Ingredients:

2 small cooked beets

1 teaspoon of pure vanilla extract

1 teaspoon of pure maple syrup

1 cup of frozen strawberries

1 cup of frozen cauliflower florets

½ cup of frozen raspberries

½ cup of frozen blueberries

2 cups of light coconut milk

½ teaspoon of ground cinnamon

2 tablespoons of unflavored collagen peptides (optional)

Preparation:

1. Beets, cauliflower, berries, coconut milk, vanilla, maple syrup, cinnamon, and collagen peptides are added to the blender (if using).
2. Blend for two minutes on high, or until completely smooth.
Recipe for 2 servings

Ingredient tips:

- Whatever frozen berries you have on hand, feel free to use them. A good source of antioxidants and dietary fiber are all berries, which will help keep you fuller, longer.
- It is strongly recommended that you add them whenever you can for their nutritional value, although the collagen peptides are optional in this recipe. Each tablespoon of collagen peptides provides 10 grams of high-quality protein which, after your morning meal, can help the gut heal and keep you full and satisfied.

Nutrients:

Calories: 318

Carb: 52g

Fiber: 9g

Fat: 13g

Protein: 6g

Wild Blueberry Coconut Milk Yogurt

Ingredients:

2 cups Creamy Coconut Milk Yogurt

¼ cup unflavored collagen peptides

2 tablespoons unsweetened shredded coconut flakes

1 cup frozen wild blueberries, thawed

2 tablespoons pure maple syrup

Preparation:

1. Combine the coconut milk yogurt, thawed blueberries, collagen peptides, maple syrup and shredded coconut in a large bowl. Mix thoroughly.
2. Divide the yogurt containing coconut milk into four serving bowls. *Recipe for 4 servings*

Ingredient tips:

- In the freezer section of your local supermarket, you can find wild blueberries. Feel free to swap out the wild blueberries for a different flavor profile for any berry you enjoy, such as raspberries or blackberries.
- In order to help heal the leaky gut, studies have shown that collagen is an important nutrient. At your local health food store or online, you can find collagen peptides.
- To save time, make this recipe ahead of time and store it all week long for easy and nutritious breakfasts in individual grab-and-go containers. For up to 5 days, refrigerate.

Nutrients:

Calories: 332

Carb: 20g

Fiber: 4g

Fat: 28g

Protein: 3g

Raspberry Cinnamon Yogurt Bowl

Ingredients:

¼ cup unsweetened coconut flakes

2 cups Creamy Coconut Milk Yogurt

2 tablespoons pure maple syrup

½ teaspoon ground cinnamon

2 cups fresh red raspberries

½ teaspoon pure vanilla extract

¼ cup unflavored collagen peptides

Preparation:

1. Toast the coconut flakes for 60 to 90 seconds in a small skillet over medium-high heat, stirring constantly, until golden brown. Just set aside.
2. Combine the coconut milk yoghurt, collagen peptides, maple syrup, vanilla, and cinnamon in a large bowl. Mix thoroughly.
3. Split the mixture into 4 bowls.
4. Use 1/2 cup of fresh red raspberries and 1 tablespoon of toasted coconut flakes to top each yogurt bowl.

Recipe for 4 servings

Ingredients tips:

- To add dietary fiber and nutrients, try diced pears or apples.
- Enjoy the cinnamon coconut yogurt as it is, or use it as a topping or filling for the Strawberry Fruit Tart for sweet treats such as Slow Cooker Poached Pears.
- In order to help heal the leaky gut, studies have shown that collagen is an important nutrient. At your local health food store or online, you can find collagen peptides.
- For no-fuss breakfasts all week long, store individual servings in grab-and-go containers, such as Mason jars. For up to 5 days, refrigerate.

Nutrients:

Calories: 318

Carb: 21g

Fiber: 7g

Fat: 26g

Protein: 3g

---

70 Coconut milk chai

Ingredient:

1 cup shredded coconut

1 vanilla bean (optional)

¾ teaspoons cinnamon

4 dates

1½-inch piece ginger

2 cups boiling water

Preparation:

1. In a high-powered blender, place all the ingredients and blend on high for a minute or two, until thoroughly mixed.
2. Let it cool down a bit and strain through a bag of cheesecloth or nut milk, taking care not to burn yourself.
3. In a saucepan, enjoy icing or reheat to serve warm.

Recipe for 1 serving

Nutrient:

Calories: 22

Carb: 8g

Fiber: 7g

Fat: 2g

Protein: 0g

STEW AND SOUPS

Fennel Apple Soup

Ingredients:

2 tablespoons extra-virgin olive oil

½ sweet onion, chopped

¼ teaspoon sea salt

1 teaspoon minced fresh garlic

2 celery stalks, chopped

1 apple (about ½ pound), peeled, cored, and diced

3 fennel bulbs, stems and fronds removed, diced

6 cups Chicken Bone Broth

1 tablespoon chopped fresh thyme or 1 teaspoon dried thyme

Preparation:

1. Over a medium heat, place a large saucepan and add the olive oil.
2. Sauté the onion and garlic for about 5 minutes, until soft and lightly browned.
3. Add the fennel bulb, celery and apple and sauté for about 8 minutes until softened.
4. Add the thyme and chicken broth and bring the soup to a boil.
5. Decrease the heat to low and simmer until the fruit and vegetables are tender, about 15 minutes.
6. Transfer the mixture to a food processor or blender, or use an immersion blender right in the pan until the soup is smooth.
7. Add salt to season and serve.

Recipe for 4 servings

Nutrient:

Calories: 182

Carb: 29g

Fiber: 7g

Fat: 7g

Protein: 3g

Sunny carrot soup

Ingredients:

2 tablespoons extra-virgin olive oil

½ sweet onion, chopped

1 tablespoon grated fresh ginger

1 teaspoon minced fresh garlic

1 teaspoon turmeric

6 cups Chicken Bone Broth (see here)

1½ pounds carrots, peeled and chopped

1 sweet potato, peeled and chopped

1 cup unsweetened organic coconut milk (for homemade, see here)

2 tablespoons freshly squeezed lemon juice

¼ teaspoon sea salt

Preparation:

1. Over a medium-high heat, place a large saucepan and add the olive oil.
2. Sauté the onion, ginger, garlic and turmeric for about 3 minutes, until the onion is soft.
3. Add the carrots, chicken broth, and sweet potato.
4. Bring the soup to a boil, then reduce the heat to low and simmer for about 20 minutes, until the carrots are tender.
5. Transfer the soup, add the coconut milk and process until the soup is smooth, to a food processor or blender.
6. To combine, add the lemon juice and salt and pulse.
7. Serve it warm.

Recipe for 4 servings

Nutrient:

Calories: 212

Carb: 33g

Fiber: 11g

Fat: 8g

Protein: 3g

French onion soup

Ingredients:

2 tablespoons coconut oil

1 tablespoon chopped fresh thyme or ½ teaspoon dried thyme

2 pounds sweet onions (about 6), halved and cut into ¼-inch slices

Juice of ½ lime

¼ teaspoon sea salt

5 cups Easy Beef Bone Broth

Preparation:

1. Over a low heat, place a large heavy-bottom saucepan and warm the coconut oil.
2. Add the onions and the thyme, stirring until the vegetables are coated in oil.
3. Cover the saucepan with a lid and allow the onions to steam for about 20 minutes, in their own juices, until they are reduced.
4. Remove the lid from the pot and continue to slowly caramelize the onions, stirring occasionally for about 90 minutes, until they are a deep caramel color.
5. To bring the soup to a simmer, add the lime juice and beef broth and raise the heat to medium.
6. Lower the heat and simmer to intensify the soup's flavor for 1 hour.
7. Add salt to season and serve.

Recipe for 4 servings

Nutrient:

Calories: 183

Carb: 28g

Fiber: 10g

Fat: 7g

Protein: 3g

Simple Borscht

Ingredients:

1 tablespoon extra-virgin olive oil

2 teaspoons minced fresh garlic

½ sweet onion, chopped

3 cups peeled and diced beets

1 cup peeled and chopped carrot

Juice of 1 lemon

1 cup shredded red cabbage

4 cups Easy Beef Bone Broth

½ teaspoon sea salt

Preparation:

1. Over a medium-high heat, place a large saucepan and add the olive oil.
2. Sauté the onion and garlic in the oil for about 3 minutes, until the vegetables are softened.
3. Add the beets, cabbage, and carrot and sauté for about 3 minutes with the vegetables.

4. Add the broth and salt to the beef and bring the soup to a boil, then reduce the heat to low and simmer for about 20 minutes until the vegetables are tender.
5. Transfer the soup to a food processor or blender, or use an immersion blender right in the saucepan and pulse until the soup is smooth.
6. Stir in the lemon juice and serve.

Recipe for 4 servings

Nutrient:

Calories: 110

Carb: 18g

Fiber: 12g

Fat: 4g

Protein: 12g

Squash-Pear Soup

Ingredients:

1 winter squash (about 3 pounds), peeled, seeded, and chopped

3 cups Chicken Bone Broth

2 pears, cored and chopped

1 teaspoon ground cinnamon

Dash ground cloves

½ teaspoon ground ginger

Dash sea salt

Preparation:

1. In a large saucepan and on medium-high heat, place the squash, pears, and chicken broth.
2. Bring the mixture to a boil and bring the heat down to low levels. Simmer for about 20 minutes, until the squash is tender.
3. Transfer the soup to a food processor or blender and process or use an immersion blender right in the saucepan until the soup is smooth.
4. To combine, add cinnamon, ginger, cloves, and salt, and pulse.
5. Serve it immediately .

Recipe for 4 servings

Nutrient:

Calories: 121

Carb: 32g

Fiber: 10g

Fat: 2g

Protein: 12g

Coconut Seafood Soup

Ingredients:

1 tablespoon extra-virgin olive oil

½ cup sliced mushrooms

1 sweet onion, chopped

1 teaspoon grated fresh ginger

¼ teaspoon sea salt

1 teaspoon minced fresh garlic

4 cups Chicken Bone Broth

1 teaspoon turmeric

½ cup peeled and shredded carrots

1 cup unsweetened organic coconut milk

3 tilapia fillets, chopped into large chunks

10 (21 to 25 count) shrimp, peeled, deveined, and each cut into 4 pieces

½ cup shredded spinach

Preparation:

1. Over a medium-high heat, place a large stockpot and add the olive oil.
2. Sauté the onion, mushrooms, garlic and ginger for about 4 minutes, until the onion is tender.
3. Add the carrots and chicken broth and bring the soup to a boil.
4. Stir in the fish, shrimp, coconut milk, turmeric and salt, and reduce the heat to a low level. Simmer the soup for about 6 minutes until the fish is fully cooked.
5. Remove the soup from the heat and stir in the spinach.
6. Serve immediately.

Recipe for 4 servings

Nutrient:

Calories: 230

Carb: 10g

Fiber: 10g

Fat: 8g

Protein: 29g

Cabbage-turkey soup

Ingredients:

2 tablespoons extra-virgin olive oil

2 teaspoons minced fresh garlic

2 cups peeled and diced carrots

1 sweet onion, chopped

6 cups shredded green cabbage (about ½ head)

1 cup chopped cooked turkey

8 cups Chicken Bone Broth

2 bay leaves

¼ teaspoon sea salt

Preparation:

1. Over a medium-high heat, place a large saucepan and add the olive oil.
2. Sauté the onion and garlic for about 3 minutes, until the onion has softened.
3. Add the carrots and cabbage. Cook for about 4 minutes to slightly soften the cabbage, stirring frequently.
4. Add the chicken broth and bay leaves, bring the soup to a boil, then reduce the heat and simmer for about 35 minutes until the vegetables are tender.
5. Add the turkey and salt and cook until the turkey is fully heated, about 5 minutes.
6. Remove and serve the bay leaves.

Recipe for 4 servings

Cauliflower bacon soup

Ingredient:

6 strips organic bacon, chopped

1 teaspoon minced fresh garlic

6 cups Chicken Bone Broth

2 leeks, whites only, chopped

2 heads cauliflower, cut into small florets

2 tablespoons chopped fresh parsley, for garnish

Preparation:

1. Fry the bacon over medium-high heat in a large saucepan, stirring frequently, until thoroughly cooked and crispy, about 5 minutes.
2. Transfer the bacon to a plate that is lined with paper towels and set aside.
3. Without wiping it out, place the saucepan back on the heat, add the leeks and garlic and sauté until softened, about 3 minutes.
4. To the saucepan, add three-fourths of the cauliflower florets and all the chicken broth. To cover the cauliflower, add a little water if the liquid isn't at least 1 inch above the vegetables.
5. Bring the soup to a boil, then reduce the heat to low and simmer for about 20 minutes, until the cauliflower is tender.
6. Place a small saucepan of water on a high heat while the soup is simmering and bring it to a boil.
7. For about 3 minutes, blanch the remaining one-fourth of the cauliflower until tender-crisp.
8. Please drain and set aside the blanched cauliflower.
9. Transfer the soup to a food processor or blender, or use an immersion blender right in the saucepan until it is smooth.
10. Add the blanched cauliflower and bacon and pour the soup back into the saucepan.
11. Serve the soup with the fresh chopped parsley garnish.
Recipe for 4 servings

Nutrient:

Calories: 152

Carb: 21g

Fiber: 7g

Fat: 5g

Protein: 6g

Vegetable and beef soup

Ingredients:

1 pound lean ground beef

1 sweet onion (diced)

3 celery stalks, diced

2 teaspoons minced fresh garlic

2 carrots, peeled and sliced into disks

1 tablespoon chopped fresh thyme or 1 teaspoon dried thyme

1 sweet potato, peeled and diced

5 cups Easy Beef Bone Broth

2 parsnips, peeled and diced

1 cup shredded cabbage

¼ teaspoon sea salt

2 tablespoons chopped fresh parsley, for garnish

Preparation:

1. Sauté the ground beef over medium-high heat in a medium stockpot until cooked, about 5 minutes.
2. Add the celery, onion and garlic, and sauté for about 4 minutes until the vegetables are tender.
3. Add the beef broth, carrots, sweet potatoes, and parsnips and bring the liquid to a simmer.
4. Lower the heat and let the soup simmer for 10 minutes.
5. Add the cabbage and thyme and simmer for about 10 minutes, until the vegetables are tender.
6. Stir the salt in.
7. Serve the fresh parsley garnished soup.

Recipe for 4 servings

Nutrient:

Calories: 340

Carb: 30g

Fiber: 8g

Fat: 7g

Protein: 37g

---

80 Savory lamb stew

Ingredients:

2 tablespoons extra-virgin olive oil

½ sweet onion, chopped

1½ pounds lamb shoulder, trimmed of visible fat and cut into 2-inch chunks

2 teaspoons minced fresh garlic

½ teaspoon ground cinnamon

1 teaspoon grated fresh ginger

½ teaspoon turmeric

¼ teaspoon ground cloves

2 cups peeled and diced carrots

2 cups Easy Beef Bone Broth

¼ teaspoon sea salt

2 tablespoons chopped fresh cilantro, for garnish

Preparation:

1. Preheat the furnace to 300°F.
2. Over medium-high heat, place a large ovenproof casserole dish on the stove top and add the olive oil.
3. Brown the lamb in the oil, stirring occasionally, for four minutes or so.
4. Add the onion, garlic, ginger, cinnamon, turmeric and cloves and sauté for about 4 minutes, until the onion is tender.
5. Bring the stew to a boil, then cover the container and place it in the oven. Add the carrots, beef broth, and salt.
6. In the oven, cook the stew until the lamb is very tender, for about 2 hours.
7. Take the stew out of the oven and serve it hot, topped with cilantro.

Recipe for 4 servings

Nutrient:

Calories: 421

Carb: 19g

Fiber: 3g

Fat: 19g

Protein: 49g

Conclusion:

Remember to pay attention to details while cooking the foods, ensure that you avoid foods that are not beneficial for healing Auto-immune diseases as we've discussed in section 2.

Choosing to adopt this protocol means consciously choosing a detoxification path thanks to a choice: CLEAN FOOD.

This road may initially seem uphill, it may seem not worth it ... after all, anyone of us thinks that food is one of the pleasures of life!!

You will have to remain lucid and focused on the final goal, because, especially the initial phase, it will be a phase of renunciation, sacrifice, and great mental test; it will be your determination, your desire to "lighten" your body from everything that is toxic for you, to bring you the physical and mental benefits. Therefore, the approach you will adopt will help you to believe in this project and to achieve the desired results.

So, why not try the AIP diet?

When deciding to adopt the Autoimmune Protocol, food choices will focus on consuming nutrients and taking dietary supplements to promote healing and provide the body with the tools and resources it needs to stop sticking and help repair damaged tissue. and then return to health.

As mentioned, a few lines above, it will not be an easy walk in the park, it will be challenging, and it will take perseverance and commitment. But following our advice to the letter, we cannot guarantee you that you will recover at all, but you will experience real benefits for your body, which will allow you to detoxify your body, and recover the joy of eating.

Our suggestions could be a way to continue to cultivate your passion for cooking (so it was for us, in creating them !!), and at the same time get closer to this protocol that is still not too well known, but which scientific studies are demonstrating its effectiveness in restoring "normality" and dignity to your life.

Keep your hunger alive in the kitchen and outside the kitchen !!

Eat clean!!

Enjoy the diet, enjoy new life!!

Your recovery begins now!!!

THANKS FOR READING!!!

Amina Subramani & Tracy Cooper

Thank you for reading this book. If you enjoyed it, please visit the site where you purchased it and write a brief review. your feedback is important to me and will help other readers decide whether to read the book too. Thank you

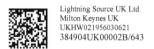

Lightning Source UK Ltd.
Milton Keynes UK
UKHW021956030621
384904UK00002B/643